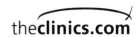

FOOT AND ANKLE CLINICS

Posttraumatic Reconstruction of the Foot and Ankle

GUEST EDITOR
Alastair S.E. Younger, MB, ChB, MSc, ChM, FRCSC

CONSULTING EDITOR
Mark S. Myerson, MD

March 2006 • Volume 11 • Number 1

SAUNDERS

An Imprint of Elsevier, Inc.
PHILADELPHIA   LONDON   TORONTO   MONTREAL   SYDNEY   TOKYO

W.B. SAUNDERS COMPANY
A Division of Elsevier Inc.

1600 John F. Kennedy Blvd., Suite 1800, Philadelphia, PA 19103-2899

http://www.theclinics.com

FOOT AND ANKLE CLINICS   Volume 11, Number 1
March 2006   ISSN 1083-7515
Editor: Debora Dellapena   ISBN 1-4160-3504-4

Reprints. For copies of 100 or more of articles in this publication, please contact the Commercial Reprints Department, Elsevier Inc., 360 Park Avenue South, New York, New York 10010-1710. Tel.: (212) 633-3813, Fax: (212) 462-1935, e-mail: reprints@elsevier.com

The ideas and opinions expressed in *Foot and Ankle Clinics* do not necessarily reflect those of the Publisher. The Publisher does not assume any responsibility for any injury and/or damage to persons or property arising out of or related to any use of the material contained in this periodical. The reader is advised to check the appropriate medical literature and the product information currently provided by the manufacturer of each drug to be administered to verify the dosage, the method and duration of administration, or contraindications. It is the responsibility of the treating physician or other health care professional, relying on independent experience and knowledge of the patient, to determine drug dosages and the best treatment for the patient. Mention of any product in this issue should not be construed as endorsement by the contributors, editors, or the Publisher of the product or manufacturers' claims.

Foot and Ankle Clinics (ISSN 1083-7515) is published quarterly by W.B. Saunders, 360 Park Avenue South, New York, NY 10010-1710. Months of publication are March, June, September, and December. Business and Editorial Offices: 1600 John F. Kennedy Blvd., Suite 1800, Philadelphia, PA 19103-2899. Accounting and Circulation Offices: 6277 Sea Harbor Drive, Orlando, FL 32887-4800. Periodicals postage paid at New York, NY, and additional mailing offices. Subscription prices are $170.00 per year for US individuals, $245.00 per year for US institutions, $85.00 per year for US students and residents, $190.00 per year for Canadian individuals, $285.00 per year for Canadian institutions, $230.00 for international individuals, $285.00 for international institutions and $110.00 per year for Canadian and foreign students residents. To receive student/resident rate, orders must be accompanied by name of affiliated institution, date of term, and the *signature* of program/residency coordinator on institution letterhead. Orders will be billed at individual rate until proof of status is received. Foreign air speed delivery is included in all *Clinics* subscription prices. All prices are subject to change without notice. POSTMASTER: Send address changes to *Foot and Ankle Clinics*, Elsevier Periodicals Customer Service, 6277 Harbor Drive, Orlando, FL 32887-4800. **Customer Service: 1-800-654-2452 (US). From outside of the US, call 1-407-345-1000.**

Printed in the United States of America.

CONSULTING EDITOR

MARK S. MYERSON, MD, President, American Orthopaedic Foot and Ankle Society; Director, The Institute for Foot and Ankle Reconstruction, Mercy Medical Center, Baltimore, Maryland

GUEST EDITOR

ALASTAIR S.E. YOUNGER, MB, ChB, MSc, ChM, FRCSC, Clinical Associate Professor, Department of Orthopaedics, The University of British Columbia, Vancouver; Director, British Columbia's Foot and Ankle Clinic, Providence Health Care, Vancouver, British Columbia, Canada

CONTRIBUTORS

ROMNEY C. ANDERSEN, MD, Staff Orthopaedic Surgeon, National Naval Medical Center, Bethesda; Assistant Professor of Surgery, Uniformed Services School of The Health Sciences, Bethesda, Maryland

JOHN G. ANDERSON, MD, Assistant Clinical Professor, Department of Orthopaedic Surgery, College of Human Medicine, Michigan State University, Grand Rapids, Michigan; Orthopaedic Associates of Grand Rapids, Foot and Ankle Division, Grand Rapids, Michigan

ROBERT B. ANDERSON, MD, Foot and Ankle Surgeon, OrthoCarolina PA, Charlotte, North Carolina

MICHAEL S. ARONOW, MD, Associate Professor, Department of Orthopaedic Surgery, University of Connecticut School of Medicine, Farmington, Connecticut

DONALD R. BOHAY, MD, Assistant Clinical Professor, Department of Orthopaedic Surgery, College of Human Medicine, Michigan State University; Orthopaedic Associates of Grand Rapids, Foot and Ankle Division, Grand Rapids, Michigan

J. CHRIS COETZEE, MD, FRCS, Associate Professor, Department of Orthopaedic Surgery, Foot and Ankle Service, University of Minnesota, Minneapolis, Minnesota

CHRISTOPHER W. DiGIOVANNI, MD, Associate Professor and Chief, Foot and Ankle Service, Department of Orthopaedic Surgery, Brown Medical School, Providence, Rhode Island

JOHN S. EARLY, MD, Texas Orthopaedic Associates LLP; Clinical Professor Orthopaedic Surgery, University of Texas Southwestern Medical Center, Dallas, Texas

JONATHAN A. FORSBERG, MD, Clinical Instructor, Uniformed Services University of the Health Sciences; Orthopaedic Resident, National Naval Medical Center, Bethesda, Maryland

MARK A. GLAZEBROOK, MD, MSc, PhD, FRCS(C), Assistant Professor, Division of Orthopedic Surgery, Dalhousie University, Halifax, Nova Scotia, Canada

TOM GOETZ, MD, FRCSC, Clinical Assistant Professor, Department of Orthopaedics, University of British Columbia, Vancouver; Providence Health Care, Vancouver, British Columbia, Canada

RENÉ GRASS, MD, PhD, Attending Trauma Surgeon, Trauma and Reconstructive Surgery, University Hospital "Carl Gustav Carus," Dresden, Germany

W. BRYCE HENDERSON, MD, FRCSC, Clinical Fellow, University Health Network–Toronto Western Hospital, University of Toronto, Toronto, Ontario, Canada

EUGENE Y. KOH, MD, PhD, Resident Surgeon, Department of Orthopaedic Surgery, Brown Medical School, Providence, Rhode Island

JOHNNY T.C. LAU, MD, MSc, FRCSC, Assistant Professor, Department of Surgery, University of Toronto; Consultant, Orthopaedic Surgeon, University Health Network–Toronto Western Hospital, Toronto, Ontario, Canada

ARTHUR MANOLI, II, MD, Director, Michigan International Foot and Ankle Center, Pontiac, Michigan

JOHN D. MASKILL, MD, Resident, Grand Rapids Medical Education and Research Center, Michigan State University Orthopaedic Surgery Residency Program, Grand Rapids, Michigan

FRANCIS X. McGUIGAN, MD, Staff Orthopaedic Surgeon, National Naval Medical Center; Associate Professor of Surgery, Uniformed Services University of the Health Sciences, Bethesda, Maryland

ANTHONY P. MECHREFE, MD, Clinical Instructor and Trauma Fellow, Department of Orthopaedic Surgery, Brown Medical School, Providence, Rhode Island

ROBERT M. MIHALICH, MD, Baylor University Medical Center, Dallas, Texas

MARK S. MYERSON, MD, President, American Orthopaedic Foot and Ankle Society; Director, The Institute for Foot and Ankle Reconstruction, Mercy Medical Center, Baltimore, Maryland

FLORIAN NICKISCH, MD, Foot and Ankle Fellow (2005–2006), OrthoCarolina PA, Charlotte, North Carolina

JUSTIN L. PALETZ, MD, FRCSC, Associate Professor, Division of Plastic Surgery, Dalhousie University, Halifax, Nova Scotia, Canada

FERNANDO A. PEÑA, MD, Assistant Professor, Department of Orthopaedic Surgery, Foot and Ankle Service, University of Minnesota, Minneapolis, Minnesota

MURRAY J. PENNER, MD, BSc(MEng), FRCSC, Clinical Assistant Professor, Division of Lower Extremity Reconstruction Foot and Ankle, Department of Orthopaedics, University of British Columbia, and British Columbia's Foot and Ankle Clinic, Vancouver, British Columbia, Canada

MARK D. PERRY, MD, Associate Professor, Department of Orthopaedic Surgery, University of Texas Southwestern Medical Center, Dallas, Texas

STEFAN RAMMELT, MD, Attending Trauma Surgeon, Trauma and Reconstructive Surgery, University Hospital "Carl Gustav Carus," Dresden, Germany

PETER G. TRAFTON, MD, FACS, Professor, Department of Orthopaedic Surgery, Brown Medical School, Providence, Rhode Island

JÖRG WINKLER, MD, Fellow in Trauma and Reconstructive Surgery, University Hospital "Carl Gustav Carus," Dresden, Germany

ALASTAIR S.E. YOUNGER, MB, ChB, MSc, ChM, FRCSC, Clinical Associate Professor, Department of Orthopaedics, The University of British Columbia, Vancouver; Director, British Columbia's Foot and Ankle Clinic, Providence Health Care, Vancouver, British Columbia, Canada

HANS ZWIPP, MD, PhD, Head of Department, Professor of Trauma Surgery, Trauma and Reconstructive Surgery, University Hospital "Carl Gustav Carus," Dresden, Germany

CONTENTS

the care of the foot and ankle should be familiar with the spectrum of injuries that concern the first ray. These injuries, their management, and sequelae are reviewed.

Foot and ankle reconstruction following blast trauma is particularly challenging based on the devastating soft tissue injuries associated with open comminuted fractures. Considering the difficulties encountered in reconstruction, the functional limitations associated with many salvaged limbs, and the superior performance of contemporary prosthetics, many injured service members may benefit more from below knee amputation than from limb salvage. Limb salvage of blast-injured extremities is a multidisciplinary effort directed toward eradication of infection, treatment of soft tissue and bone defects, and management of late reconstructive procedures. External ring fixators have an important and expanding role in the treatment algorithm.

Nerve injuries of the foot and ankle can result in pain, numbness, or loss of motor function. A thorough history and physical examination are required to diagnose the injury correctly and guide treatment. Treatment may involve conservative measures, primary nerve repair or nerve grafting, or resection and relocation of painful neuroma. Potential complications include the development of chronic pain syndromes.

Compartment syndrome should be treated early and aggressively to prevent late complications. Patients may have late deformity because of a failure of diagnosis, inadequate decompression, or a delay in fasciotomies. Late reconstruction will allow a plantigrade and relatively functional foot. Complete excision of scarred muscle will prevent recurrence in established deformities. Early treatment may prevent significant functional impairment by well-placed tenotomies. In patients with severe long-term deformities with extensive soft tissue contraction, incremental correction may be an appropriate intermediate intervention.

FORTHCOMING ISSUES

June 2006
Arthroscopy and Endoscopy of the Foot and Ankle
Niek van Dijk, MD, *Guest Editor*

September 2006
Instability and Impingement Syndrome
Nicola Maffulli, MD, MS, PhD, FRCS(Orth), *Guest Editor*

December 2006
The Diabetic Foot and Ankle
Brian G. Donley, MD, *Guest Editor*

RECENT ISSUES

December 2005
Orthobiologics
Sheldon S. Lin, MD, *Guest Editor*

September 2005
The Calcaneus
Paul J. Juliano, MD, *Guest Editor*

June 2005
Achilles Tendon
Nicola Maffulli, MD, MS, PhD, FRCS(Orth), *Guest Editor*

THE CLINICS ARE NOW AVAILABLE ONLINE!

http://www.theclinics.com

FOOT AND
ANKLE CLINICS

Foot Ankle Clin N Am
11 (2006) xiii

Preface

Posttraumatic Reconstruction of the Foot and Ankle

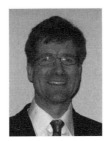

Alastair S.E. Younger, MB, ChB, MSc, ChM, FRCSC
Guest Editor

Posttraumatic deformities of the foot and ankle continue to challenge any surgeon willing to take on these complex cases. Often the initial treatment will create problems for the surgeon, making these cases some of the most complex to address.

I am fortunate as Guest Editor to have so many talented authors contributing to this issue of the *Foot and Ankle Clinics of North America*. The first articles address issues from an anatomic viewpoint, starting proximally and working distally. The final articles address more generic issues such as soft tissue coverage, nerve injuries, and treatment of infection. The article by Dr. McGuigan and colleagues outlines some of the injuries that may need to be reconstructed by surgeons seeing veterans of present conflicts.

I hope that by reading this issue, you learn as much as I did by editing it.

Alastair S.E. Younger, MB, ChB, MSc, ChM, FRCSC
Department of Orthopaedics
The University of British Columbia
401-1160 Burrard Street
Vancouver, BC V6Z 2E8, Canada
E-mail address: asyounger@shaw.ca

1083-7515/06/$ – see front matter © 2006 Elsevier Inc. All rights reserved.
doi:10.1016/j.fcl.2006.01.002

ELSEVIER
SAUNDERS

Foot Ankle Clin N Am
11 (2006) 1–18

FOOT AND
ANKLE CLINICS

Tibial Nonunion

Anthony P. Mechrefe, MD, Eugene Y. Koh, MD, PhD,
Peter G. Trafton, MD, Christopher W. DiGiovanni, MD*

*Department of Orthopaedic Surgery, Brown Medical School, Rhode Island Hospital,
1287 North Main Street, Providence, RI 02903, USA*

Because some tibial fractures will fail to heal, the surgeon must forewarn the patient of this possibility. Patients who have a tibial fracture must be followed carefully so that timely intervention can be offered if bone healing fails to progress. Slow functional recovery and persistent disabling pain at the fracture site are reliable clues to nonunion. Operative treatment is safe and effective for tibial nonunions but not without risk. Numerous treatment options exist. Surgeons should be familiar with several treatment options. Surgeons should identify the delayed bone healing and establish the need for management by referring the patient to an expert in the care of nonunions. Reasonably aligned, aseptic nonunions generally respond to surgery that is designed to increase their stability or the augmentation of their healing response with bone graft. Management of infected nonunions is more challenging.

Symptomatic tibial nonunions result in significant disability and loss of function. The surgeon must address the orthopedic issues as well as the psychosocial, family, and work issues constraints that prevent recovery. The problems that face a patient who suffers from a tibial nonunion include pain control, narcotic dependence, lost work, lost wages, failed treatment plans, prolonged treatment, inadequate mobility, and the possibility of amputation [1]. The intense and lengthy time course that is required for treating tibial nonunions can be costly to the patient, their family, and the surgeon.

* Corresponding author.
E-mail address: yodigi@aol.com (C.W. DiGiovanni).

Definition/classification

A small percentage of tibial shaft fractures fail to unite within an appropriate time after injury. Healing times vary from 6 to 9 months, but any time limit is arbitrary. Factors that affect bone healing include injury severity, local infection, smoking, and other patient comorbidities. A tibial shaft fracture nonunion is one that fails to show progressive radiographic healing over 3 consecutive months. The classic radiographic appearance of nonunion—a distinct gap between sclerotic, hypertrophic, or atrophic bone ends—is a late finding. A nonunion is likely to cause ongoing pain before it is apparent radiographically. A nonunion may cause hardware failure–an event that may imply nonunion. A delayed union indicates that fracture healing is anticipated given enough time; the surgeon defers significant additional treatment. Although some heal, prolonged deferral of treatment results in ongoing disability until surgical intervention and recovery results in union and improved function. Proactive treatment reduces the recovery time.

Nonunions are divided into those with significant local bone formation (hypertrophic) and those that lack new bone (atrophic). An intermediate classification—oligotrophic nonunion—behaves like hypertrophic nonunions. Hypertrophic nonunions have a rich local vascular network with preservation of osteogenesis and healing potential. These fractures heal if their mechanical environment is made more stable. Neither bone graft nor debridement of the nonunion site is required. Atrophic nonunions show minimal bone formation at the fracture ends. Although this has been ascribed to poor local blood supply, histologic studies do not confirm a lack of blood vessels. Regardless, atrophic nonunions have suppressed local osteogenesis [2]. In addition to providing an optimal mechanical environment, atrophic nonunions require bone grafting or other biologic supplementation to induce osteogenesis. Typically, they exhibit indolent-appearing scar tissue between the two ends of the fracture. Surgical repair involves removal of this tissue, and apposition of the visibly viable (bleeding) bone ends. If a true late pseudarthrosis has developed, there is a false joint with a fluid-filled cavity between the bone ends. This tissue must be resected back to bleeding bone, stabilized, and grafted. In addition to deficient healing with or without callus, the alignment and stability of the nonhealed fracture must be assessed. Infection can affect treatment and prognosis and may cause the nonunion. Infection may be grossly evident or occult at the nonunion site and always must be excluded in a tibial nonunion.

Fracture healing

To treat nonunions, the biologic and mechanical aspects of bone healing must be considered [3]. Fracture repair includes cell recruitment, osteoinduction, and osteoconduction. The recruitment phase results in osteoprogenitor cells migrating to the fracture site. In the osteoinductive phase, the osteoprogenitor cells differentiate into osteoblasts secondary to local factors. In the final osteoconduction phase, bone production results in fracture stability. Surgical stabilization at the fracture site by intramedullary fixation in the tibia allows bone bridging callus formation—a process that closely resembles endochondral bone formation. Alternatively, compression at the fracture site with lag screws or compression plating provides absolute stability, and leads to direct healing without callus formation (primary bone healing). All fracture sites require mechanical stability and enough blood supply to the cells to create a healing cascade. Different fixation constructs have differential effects on mechanical stability and preservation of blood supply. External fixation maximizes blood supply but provides less mechanical stability. Rigid compressive plate and screw fixation provides absolute stability at the cost of some diminished blood supply. The fracture type, location, and associated soft tissue injuries as well as surgeon expertise may affect the choice of fixation. Loss of mechanical stability or blood supply results in a higher chance of nonunion.

Etiology/risk factors

A tibial nonunion has many causes. Chatziyiannakis and colleagues [4] showed that open fractures, soft tissue injury, increased comminution, soft tissue stripping at surgery, and a fracture of the ipsilateral fibula may increase the nonunion rate. Infection at the fracture site (associated with open fractures) contributes to nonunion [1,5]. The vascular status at the time of injury affects fracture outcome. A concomitant vascular injury increases nonunion rates by threefold [6–8]. Arterial injuries double the rate of osteomyelitis, and hence, infected nonunions [7]. Smoking contributes to delayed union and nonunion [9,10] and doubles the time for fracture healing [10]. Animal studies confirm the detrimental effects of nicotine on bone healing [9], with an increased risk of nonunion and weaker callus formation. Risk factors for nonunion include patient medications (calcium channel blocker, nonsteroidal anti-inflammatory drugs [NSAIDs], and steroids), renal insufficiency, vascular insufficiency, and smoking [11]. Preservation of tibial blood supply improves bone healing. Loss of tibial blood supply may be secondary to pharmacologic vasoconstriction and traumatic and iatrogenic periosteal stripping.

Diagnosis

Patients who have ununited tibial shaft fractures have persistent or worsening pain at the fracture site. Physical examination demonstrates tenderness (worse on stress), swelling, and warmth at the fracture site. The diagnostic work-up should include a thorough review of the patient's history. Open wounds, the severity of the trauma, difficulties with wound healing, antibiotic treatment, and sinus tracts or drainage indicate septic nonunions. Review of nonsurgical management and previous operative reports and radiographs complete the assessment. Two views of the tibia (anteroposterior [AP] and lateral) are adequate for identifying the presence and location of nonunion. Occasionally, 45° internal and external oblique views may demonstrate a nonunion in an oblique plane. Fluoroscopy can identify the correct plane of the nonunion. Stress views may demonstrate unstable nonunions.

MRI and CT scanning are useful in certain situations. These studies and their interpretation may be unreliable in diagnosing nonunions. The presence of hardware may obscure the nonunion. Newer techniques and software suppress metal artifact and improve the diagnostic accuracy of the study. Radionuclide scanning can evaluate nonunions and osteomyelitis. The scan confirms increased bone turnover from any cause. Bone scans (technectium-99m diphosphonate or gallium-67 citrate) are "hot" when viable bone is not united. In a true pseudoarthrosis, a bone scan is cold in the center of a nonunion. They are unable to differentiate adequately between healing bone and subclinical infection. Indium-111–labeled leukocyte scans detect osteomyelitis and yield false positive and false negative results, particularly with indolent bone infection [12]. A tissue biopsy is a valuable tool for ruling out infection as a potential inhibitor of fracture repair. To improve diagnostic accuracy, the patient should be off all antibiotics and multiple samples should be obtained. Aerobic, anaerobic, fungal, and acid-fast cultures detect the wide spectrum of infectious organisms that can inhibit fracture healing. Histopathology can assist in diagnosing infection and rule out other pathology. Careful surgical technique in taking these samples should be used. Sedimentation rate and c-reactive protein are useful markers in diagnosing musculoskeletal infection. A white cell scan, however, has little diagnostic accuracy because it lacks specificity [13].

Often the diagnosis of an ununited tibial shaft fracture requires surgical exploration, with direct visual confirmation of motion at the fracture site. There is almost always a single plane in which motion occurs. No other test reliably establishes the diagnosis of failure to unite. Patients should understand that the final diagnosis may be obtained at the time of surgery.

Treatment options

When planning treatment for a patient who has a tibial nonunion, the surgeon must determine if the nonunion is symptomatic. The patient's pain and dysfunction are determined. The degree of disability and its duration are assessed. Interference with work, and social and recreational activities is recorded. A patient may not be troubled enough by an ununited tibia fracture to warrant significant treatment, as long as he is able to manage necessary activities. If the patient is symptomatic, the surgeon must confirm that the symptoms are due to the nonunion by localizing and correlating the pain to the nonunion site.

If significant deformity is present at the nonunion site correction must be obtained. If the nonunion is mobile, the deformity is corrected by indirect manipulation. This must be assessed carefully, usually with intraoperative radiographs. A successful realignment still may not permit passage of an intramedullary nail. If the deformity is too stiff for this correction, the nonunion will require surgical excision and fixation with plate or nail, if the local soft tissues are adequate. A poor soft tissue envelope may require tissue coverage procedures or Ilizarov external fixation with bone transport, deformity correction, and traction-compression.

Instability of an ununited tibia fracture causes disability and discomfort during activity. Stable, well-aligned nonunions can be treated nonoperatively if their impact on the patient's comfort and function is tolerable. External bracing can be used occasionally to support an unstable, ununited tibial shaft fracture and achieve function and comfort levels that are acceptable to a sedentary patient. Bone healing may be stimulated by magnetic fields or ultrasound. Generally, most unstable nonunions require surgical repair to gain union in a satisfactory position. Because most mobile nonunions are atrophic, consideration also should be given to bone grafting. Weight-bearing activity also is believed to stimulate healing. A "bone stimulator" is a reasonable treatment option. The decision whether to proceed with surgical management depends upon symptoms.

The presence of any retained internal fixation is assessed. Most tibial shaft fractures are treated acutely with intramedullary nails. A well-aligned, non-infected, nailed tibial fracture should heal in 6 months. Small-diameter "unreamed" nails and their smaller locking screws may bend and break from repetitive loading before the fracture heals. This makes hardware removal difficult. Larger nails and locking screws are less likely to fracture, but if the bone fails to heal they may loosen in the bone or fracture eventually. Most tibial fractures that do not heal after intramedullary nailing will do so after "nail exchange." The existing nail is removed, the medullary canal is reamed, and a larger nail is inserted. Bone grafting usually is not required unless the original fracture was open and bone was lost from the fracture site [14,15]. Occasionally, nail exchange must be repeated if it does not work the first time. Nail exchange requires limited surgical intervention without direct fracture site exposure or bone graft harvest, and rapid return to weight bearing.

A tibia fracture that originally was treated with a plate may develop a nonunion with hardware failure but still have good alignment. In such cases, hardware removal may permit insertion of an intramedullary nail with early weight bearing and durable fixation that can outlast slowly progressive healing. Patients who have healing problems after external fixation present with late loss of alignment and painful nonunion after external fixator removal. These patients may have a history of pin site infections. If surgical repair is required, plate fixation or the use of an external fixator should be considered because of the risk of infection after intramedullary nailing, which likely is related to bacterial persistence perhaps from previous open fracture wound or pin site contamination. Hypertrophic nonunions, often with mild angulation, can be seen after primary external fixation or after initial nonoperative treatment. They have little, if any, palpable mobility; however, their deformity usually can be corrected by applying a tension-band plate on the convex side of the callus, which typically loads this sufficiently to correct angulation intraoperatively. Hypertrophic nonunions that are treated this way heal almost always and permit resumption of weight bearing. Because of their dense intramedullary callus, it is difficult to use an intramedullary nail. The presence of such callus should be anticipated whenever the surgeon chooses to nail a nonunion that was treated previously by external fixation, a plate, or a cast.

The surgeon must determine whether the ununited tibial shaft fracture is infected. Obvious physical examination findings of inflammation or a persistent sinus may be present. There may be no evidence of active infection at the time of evaluation. The patient may have a history of infection. If infection is present or suspected, treatment must begin with debridement and multiple bone and deep tissue samples taken for culture. This step establishes the diagnosis of infection and assists in appropriate antibiotic choice. When infection is present, definitive repair may be delayed and provisional stabilization with an external fixator is performed in conjunction with the first-stage debridement. External fixation should be applied to allow access to the wound for multiple debridements and flap coverage if needed. The patient who has an infected nonunion requires individualized treatment. Infection can recur around hardware, particularly with an intramedullary nail. If the fracture has healed securely, removal of the nail, gentle reaming to debride the medullary canal, and another course of culture-based antibiotics usually result in long-term infection control.

Surgical attempts to reconstruct an ununited tibia in patients who exhibit severe or prolonged debility may not be in their best interests. If the nonunion is infected, the nearby joints are stiff, or the limb is deformed and the patient has endured multiple previous salvage attempts, then amputation may provide a faster recovery and better outcome. Multiple operative attempts to gain union increase the risk of failure for subsequent surgery. Systemic factors, such as smoking, atherosclerosis, diabetes mellitus, HIV/AIDS, hepatitis C, or immunosuppression after organ transplant, affect treatment adversely. Because nonunion surgery is elective there should be adequate time for careful evaluation, preoperative planning, and consultation or referral as appropriate.

Nonoperative treatment

Previously, braces were used for patients who had ununited tibia shaft fractures primarily to restore function. Many of these patients healed slowly while they walked and worked in weight-bearing braces. Sarmiento and colleagues [16] provided much support for modern functional bracing as treatment for properly chosen nonunions. For the patient who has acceptable alignment, comfort, and function, or the individual who wishes not to proceed with surgery, functional bracing is an alternative. A custom-fitted brace that allows the use of a comfortable walking shoe probably is optimal. Unless the fracture is distal, ankle motion in the brace does not compromise bony stability.

Various adjunctive treatments may stimulate bone healing [17]. In the 1970s, Basset and colleagues [18] used electromagnetic fields to promote bone healing. Ito and Shirai [19] reported an 83% success rate of healing nonunions with electrical stimulation. Treatment failures occurred in atrophic nonunions secondary to poor blood supply at the nonunion site. These investigators concluded that electromagnetic therapy was most beneficial to hypertrophic, but not atrophic, nonunions. Low-intensity pulsed ultrasound followed as a means of extraskeletal bone stimulation. Mayr and colleagues [11] reported a success rate of 91% for delayed unions and 86% for nonunions in a wide variety of bones, including tibial nonunions. Extracorporeal shock wave therapy has been suggested as a noninvasive treatment but remains unproven [20].

These techniques may promote bone healing for some patients. They do not restore alignment or fill in bone defects. Their effectiveness is compromised by fracture motion. Bone stimulation may assist surgical repair, which by itself is more effective than any bone stimulator. It seems reasonable to limit the use of stimulators to patients who have ununited tibial fractures with acceptable alignment and who wish to defer surgery. Low-energy ultrasound may accelerate the healing of nonoperatively treated acute tibial shaft fractures, particularly in smokers, but it is not helpful when added to intramedullary nail fixation of more severe fractures [3].

Surgical treatment for aseptic nonunions

A detailed preoperative plan should take into consideration the location and classification of nonunion; the fracture deformity and stability; the patency of the medullary canal; and previous treatment, including retained hardware. Radiographic studies are used to determine the alignment and patency of the medullary canal if intramedullary nailing is planned. Radiodense bone may be avascular and requires debridement. The soft tissue envelope is examined for previous free flaps, soft tissue grafts, the position of neurovascular structures, and previous infection to plan the surgical treatment and approach. Septic nonunions may require staged intervention to control the infection and treat nonunion. Aseptic nonunions can be treated with single-stage intervention unless reconstruction of severely compromised soft tissue is required.

Bone grafting

Bone grafting is indicated for atrophic nonunions to enhance osteoinduction and osteoconduction. Cortical bone graft can provide mechanical stabilization of the nonunion. Generally, it is not warranted in hypertrophic nonunions. The gold standard for atrophic nonunions is cancellous autograft, obtained from the anterior or posterior iliac crest or the ipsilateral Gerdy's tubercle. Anteromedial and posterolateral approaches for the application of harvested bone graft have been reported [21]. For proximal third tibial nonunions, an anteromedial or postero-medial approach is favored. For distal tibial nonunions, the posterolateral approach avoids the thin soft tissue over the anteromedial tibia. Subperiosteal dissection should be avoided. An osteotome or chisel is used to lift thin strips of cortex with periosteum attached to create a vascular bed for bone graft. This "shingling" or osteoperiosteal petalling preserves periosteal blood flow to the elevated bone fragments, and provides a well-vascularized bed for additional bone graft. The soft tissues are left in continuity with the bone to provide vascularity.

Other methods for bone grafting include tibiofibular synostosis [22,23], free vascularized bone grafts [24,25], and fibula–pro-tibia grafting [26]. Autologous bone graft between tibia and fibula may promote tibiofibular synostosis [22]. Rijnberg and van Linge [23] used autogenous iliac crest bone to create a bridge between the tibia and fibula at the site of the nonunion (tibiofibular synostosis). They reported a 93% success rate in treating infected and aseptic tibial non-unions. For posterolateral grafting, corticocancellous bone chips work more effectively with a shorter healing time than does a whole iliac crest graft or a nonvascularized fibular graft [22]. This method is useful for tibial nonunions with short segmental defects. Free vascularized bone grafts are used for infected tibial nonunions (see later discussion) [24,25]. They are prone to late mechanical fail-ure and require stable fixation with additional autologous bone [24,25]. The fibula–pro-tibia technique involves fusion of the tibia and fibula, with or without medial transfer of the fibula [26].

A less invasive technique that uses percutaneous harvest and injection of autologous bone marrow into the nonunion is an alternative to bone graft for inducing osteogenesis [27,28]. Garg and colleagues [27] reported an 85% success rate of healing nonunions. Concentrating the bone marrow to maximize the number of osteogenic stem cells by a centrifuge may improve the union rate [28]. The relative efficacy of autologous bone marrow compared with bone graft remains uncertain.

Biologic supplementation

Bone morphogenic protein (BMP) can be extracted from bone and used to stimulate bone formation in soft tissue or to promote bone healing [29]. These growth factors are promoters of osteogenesis. OP-1 (osteogenic protein–1) (Stryker Biotech, Hopkinton, Massachusetts), initially describes as BMP-7, and BMP-2 (Infuse, Medtronics, Minneapolis, Minnesota), are available for clinical use [30,31]. For tibial nonunions, OP-1 and autogenous bone graft have similar outcomes [30]. The group that was treated with OP-1 had fewer infections, lower operative blood loss, and better pain control. In treating open fractures, a similar protein from the same family (BMP-2) was used during initial management of open tibial fractures that were stabilized with intramedullary nail fixation [31]. Patients who were treated with BMP-2 had fewer nonunions, fewer hardware failures, and reduced infection rates. BMP-7 and BMP-2 seem to be promising alternatives to autologous grafts. Preliminary results with these proteins are encouraging and their application (aside from cost) carries the potential for easy, rapid, at-site delivery without any donor site morbidity. This technology seems to provide an effective alternative to autologous bone graft. Prospective, randomized, controlled trials are necessary to determine its role.

Methods of fixation

Three main options exist for mechanical stabilization of tibial nonunions: intramedullary nail fixation, plate fixation, and external fixation [3]. Intramedullary nailing is a percutaneous surgical procedure; however, in the event of infection the entire medullary canal may be contaminated [32]. External fixation is the least invasive and should be considered for patients who have poor soft tissue envelopes. A stable Ilizarov ring fixator can be used for progressive correction of deformity, for transport of bone through a defect, and for mechanically altering the fracture site to stimulate union. An Ilizarov frame permits weight bearing, but might need to be in place for many months. Hypertrophic nonunions require stability for successful healing. A plate applied as a tension band, using the Arbeitsgemeinschaft für Osteosynthesefragen external tension device, is an elegant way to provide stability and correct deformity, because hypertrophic callus usually is deformable. Intramedullary nailing is technically difficult for hypertrophic nonunions, and should be avoided unless an established medullary canal is present. Plates can be used as compression or as bridge plates to stabilize nonunions, and can be augmented with bone graft to optimize bone healing. During intramedullary nail fixation, the process of reaming perturbs the endosteal blood supply, and a compensatory increase from the periosteal blood supply ensues. The additional blood supply often stimulates sufficient bone healing, thereby eliminating the need to utilize bone graft supplements (Fig. 1).

Intramedullary exchange nailing

Exchange nailing is the most convenient and effective treatment for patients who have tibia fracture nonunions after primary intramedullary nailing [14,15,33]. No significant deformity can be obtained. Removal of the nail is guided by old operative reports. The canal is reamed an additional 2 to 4 mm in diameter, and a larger diameter nail—at least 2 mm greater than the former—is inserted. Reaming (without a tourniquet) stimulates bone formation by temporarily disturbing the endosteal blood supply and eliciting a compensatory perios-

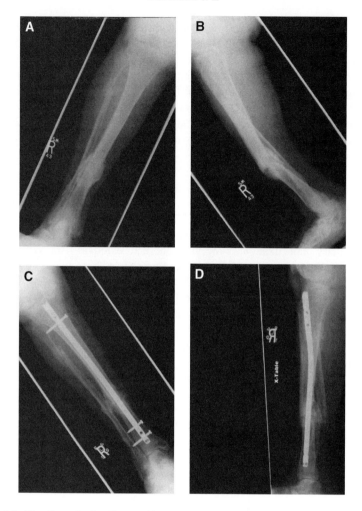

Fig. 1. (*A*) AP radiograph of a 40-year-old man who had a tibial nonunion that was treated with a fracture brace. (*B*) Lateral radiograph of tibial nonunion. (*C*) AP radiograph after intramedullary nail fixation of tibial shaft nonunion. (*D*) Lateral radiograph demonstrating healed tibial nonunion.

teal vascular reaction. The intramedullary nail is locked in the shorter segment to ensure angular and rotational stability. The opposite end is stabilized dynamically to allow weight-bearing compression at the nonunion site. The reamings are cultured to detect subclinical infection. Whether adding a fibulectomy improves the results of exchange nailing has not been determined [34]. Caution is advised when exchange nailing is selected for previous open fractures, particularly grade IIIB fractures, because there is an increased risk for infection and nonunion [14,35].

If an intramedullary nail is considered for a tibial nonunion that was not nailed previously, the surgeon should assess the previous method of fixation and plan an approach for removal, if needed. A nonpatent medullary canal may prevent insertion of an intramedullary nail or require open debridement to do so. The alignment of the nonunion may prevent reduction and passage of the nail or may require direct exposure and reduction. If the tibia was plated, plate removal may be required. Cultures should be obtained. Fibulotomy may be necessary to realign the tibia and should be done at a different level.

If external fixation was used, the fixator pins may contaminate the tibial canal. Intramedullary nailing may spread and propagate the infection [36]. Medullary callus that obstructs the canal can be perforated with a "Kuntscher pseudarthrosis chisel" (stout, but malleable sharp guidepin) or hand reamers under fluoroscopic guidance. Occasionally, the nonunion needs to be exposed through an open procedure. Then a drill can be utilized to perforate the callus. Different from acute fractures, nonunions may benefit from dynamic nail locking, and early weight bearing to promote compressive loading as a mechanical stimulus for fracture healing. The fracture site may need to be opened to restore alignment, add bone graft, and occasionally, to ensure adequate cultures.

Plate fixation

Tension-band plate fixation is an effective means of repairing tibial shaft hypertrophic nonunions, as long as the overlying soft tissue is healthy. Tension-band plating provides deformity correction and compression at the nonunion site if applied to the convex side. Helfet and colleagues [37] used tension-band plating to treat malaligned diaphyseal tibial nonunions that were not amenable to intramedullary nailing. All 33 nonunions healed, with deformity correction in 32 out of 33 patients.

Because of the wound complications, plate fixation is indicated primarily when the medullary canal is not amenable to intramedullary nailing. Other indications include the need for deformity correction and previous external fixation. There is a lower risk for infection using plate fixation compared with intramedullary nailing with previous long-term external fixation [36]. The surrounding soft tissue and periosteum should be preserved. Cancellous bone grafting should be added for atrophic nonunions. If there is inadequate soft tissue coverage a transferred muscle flap is required and a preoperative plastic surgery consultation can be invaluable.

If adequate bony apposition is obtained, the site should be stabilized with compression plating or with lag screws and neutralization plate fixation (Fig. 2). A plate may bridge a gap and the defect can be filled with autologous graft, assuming that a well-vascularized bed is present. If the defect is more than 5 cm, bone transport is preferable to plating [38,39]. The plate that is used to repair a tibial shaft nonunion should be long enough to provide stable proximal and distal fixation. A blade plate can be used for fixation close to the knee or ankle joint [40–42]. Reed and colleagues [42] used a precontoured cannulated blade plate

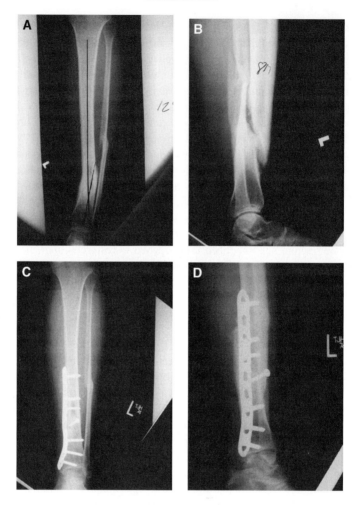

Fig. 2. (*A*) AP radiograph of a 26-year-old woman who had a tibial nonunion that was treated with functional bracing for 18 months. (*B*) Lateral radiograph of tibial malunion. (*C*) AP radiograph after reduction, bone grafting, and plating of tibial shaft nonunion. (*D*) Lateral radiograph of healed tibial nonunion after reduction and plating.

supplemented with bone grafting through a posteromedial approach. Blade plating seems to be a valid option for treating tibia metaphyseal nonunions.

External fixators and Ilizarov techniques

In addition to the techniques of open plating and intramedullary nailing, external fixators may be chosen to treat tibial nonunions as either a temporizing measure or the definitive treatment. The external fixator may be used as temporary stabilization in the event of infection or if there is poor soft tissue coverage.

For definitive treatment, the external fixator must provide adequate stability and be left in place until the bone is healed. Typically, the external fixator may be supplemented with bone graft or replaced with internal fixation (Fig. 3). Ilizarov distraction histogenesis has been used effectively for bone loss of greater than 2 cm, especially when infection is present. Angular deformity can be corrected. The outcome is determined by the surgeon's experience. Ilizarov treatment requires prolonged external fixation with careful monitoring, frame adjustments, pin site care, and occasional supplementary bone grafting. The technique is taxing for the patient and surgeon. Kabata and colleagues [43] reported the

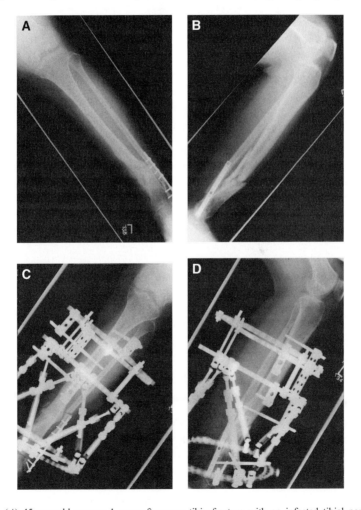

Fig. 3. (*A*) 45-year-old woman 1 year after open tibia fracture with an infected tibial nonunion. (*B*) Lateral radiograph demonstrating tibial nonunion. (*C*) AP radiograph after debridement of infected tibia and application of Taylor spatial frame (TSF). (*D*) Lateral radiograph with TSF in place. (*E*) AP radiograph of healed infected nonunion after removal of TSF. (*F*) Lateral radiograph of healed infected tibial nonunion.

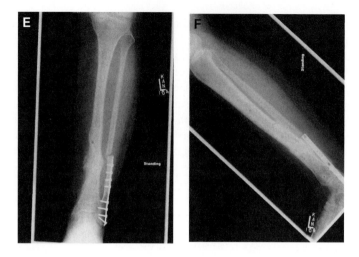

Fig. 3 (*continued*).

effective use of Ilizarov fixators with bone transport to treat juxta-articular nonunions with bone loss and malalignment of the distal femur, proximal tibia, and distal tibia. Two of the seven patients in this series had intramedullary nailing in combination with external fixation to decrease the duration of the external fixation.

Surgical treatment for infected nonunions

Infected nonunions are challenging and extremely difficult orthopedic problems [3,44]. The infection should be controlled and the nonunion healed. The nature of the infection dictates the initial treatment strategy. The virulence of the infecting organism and overall patient health must be taken into account when considering prognosis. Infected nonunions are quiescent or active [44,45]. Quiescent infected nonunions may have a history of infection and a positive bone scan, but no drainage for 3 months. Quiescent infected nonunions can be treated like noninfected nonunions, with external or internal fixation. Providing mechanical stabilization aids in eradicating the infection and promotes the healing of the nonunion [44,46]. Compression alone at the nonunion site with external fixation may be enough to eliminate the quiescent infection [47].

Cierny and colleagues [5,48] categorized actively infected nonunions by anatomic location (medullary, superficial, localized, and diffuse) and immune competency of the host (A, B, and C) with the risk of infection increasing with reduced host resistance. This classification scheme aids in the planning of debridement, based on how much bone is involved. Patients who have active infections require formal debridement with removal of all necrotic soft tissue and bone and all hardware, drainage of abscesses, and the acquisition of intra-operative cultures. Infections may require serial debridements. With such extensive debridement, the wound may require a flap for soft tissue, bone, or hardware coverage. Such plastic surgery should be delayed until debridement is adequate and infection is under control. Alternatively, a vacuum-assisted closure can promote wound healing by secondary intention [49]. The use of antibiotic-impregnated polymethyl methacrylate (PMMA) beads also can provide a temporary dressing (eg, with tobramycin or vancomycin), which is covered with an adherent plastic dressing [50]. Bead pouches provide a high local dose of antibiotics while preventing tissue desiccation and contamination. PMMA beads can serve as temporary space fillers that are replaced later with bone graft, which avoids graft placement into an infected wound. McKee and colleagues [51] used bioabsorbable, tobramycin-impregnated bone graft substitute pellets to help eradicate infections in nonunions. They reported a 92% success rate in eliminating infection, but more than 50% of the nonunions required subsequent autologous bone grafting.

After the infection has been controlled with surgical and pharmacologic means, the nonunion must be treated. For bone defects that are less than 3 to 4 cm, autologous cancellous bone or corticocancellous bone heals the defect if the fracture also is stabilized. Allografts are not appropriate in this setting. Jain and Sinha [44] developed an algorithm for treating infected nonunions of long bones. Treatment was stratified based on whether the nonunion was quiescent or actively infected. For quiescent infections with bone gaps that are smaller than 4 cm, a simple one-stage procedure with bone grafting and fracture stabilization provided good outcome. For active infections with bone gaps that were smaller than 4 cm, a two-stage procedure was used with adequate debridement and fracture stabilization, with bone grafting at a later stage. For active and quiescent infected nonunions with bone gaps that were greater than 4 cm, Ilizarov bone transport was used. Alternatively, a vascularized fibular graft can be used [25,52]. Yajima and colleagues [52] used the vascularized fibular grafting to treat nonunions that were infected with methicillin-resistant *Staphylococcus aureus*. Although they reported a 90% success rate of healing the nonunion, approximately 30% of the patients had recurrences of the infection. Late mechanical graft failure, perhaps related to insufficient use, makes free-vascular fibula grafting a less attractive option. Questionable patency of anterior and posterior tibial vessels or large areas of scarring and skin loss are relative contraindications to vascularized fibular grafting [53]. For large tibial defects with recalcitrant infected nonunions, the Ilizarov technique, or similarly the Taylor spatial frame (Smith & Nephew, Memphis, Tennessee) can be utilized (see Fig. 3). Patients who need such treatments are rare in most trauma-reconstructive practices.

If the patient has failed numerous operations, endured serious complications, and suffered repeated reinfections that have compromised severely his/her function or ability to enjoy life over a substantial time period, or if the patient obviously lacks the ability to heal or combat infection based on host factors, then the surgeon and patient may elect for an amputation. Given recent advances in prosthetics, the recovery from amputation may represent the fastest exit from the hospital setting, return to social and work environments, and reintegration into a more normal quality of life [1]. Although amputation is a valuable means of salvaging difficult infected nonunion cases, it must be considered and presented as a positive reconstructive procedure for the patient who is dealing with this difficult disease.

Summary

Tibial nonunions are complex, challenging problems for the surgeon and patient. A careful assessment of each patient's problems is required to plan an optimally effective treatment program. Crucial elements of managing a tibial nonunion include determining the presence or absence of infection and whether the nonunion is hypertrophic or atrophic. Host factors that preclude healing also may require treatment. The optimal means of stabilizing the fracture site (open internal fixation, intramedullary nailing, or external fixation) should be determined. The need for bone graft or alternatives, and the presence of any other issues that may affect outcome (eg, malalignment correction, soft tissue status, previous hardware that requires attention) must be evaluated. Finally, some patients might be more appropriate candidates for amputation. In most cases, the type and anatomy of the ununited fracture determines the treatment strategy. Atrophic nonunions usually require bone grafting in addition to mechanical stabilization, whereas hypertrophic nonunions usually heal with only mechanical stabilization. Often, the more complicated infected nonunions are treated in a staged fashion to eradicate infection and to achieve bony union. Treatment of patients who have tibial nonunion often requires attention to many nontechnical aspects of care, such as pain control, psychosocial issues, and economic issues. It also must be remembered that when these patients present, they usually are distressed by the length of their recovery. Thus, counseling about realistic timelines and outcome expectations cannot be ignored. Future management of these problems may become easier, or even unnecessary, with the advent of recombinant DNA technology, tissue engineering, and biologic agents that are designed to promote local bone growth. These technologies may improve our ability to prevent and treat tibial fracture nonunions significantly.

References

[1] Toh CL, Jupiter JB. The infected nonunion of the tibia. Clin Orthop Relat Res 1995;315: 176–91.
[2] Reed AA, Joyner CJ, Isefuku S, et al. Vascularity in a new model of atrophic nonunion. J Bone Joint Surg Br 2003;85:604–10.
[3] Rodriguez-Merchan EC, Forriol F. Nonunion: general principles and experimental data. Clin Orthop Relat Res 2004;Feb(419):4–12.
[4] Chatziyiannakis AA, Verettas DA, Raptis VK, et al. Nonunion of tibial fractures treated with

external fixation. Contributing factors studied in 71 fractures. Acta Orthop Scand Suppl 1997; 275:77–9.

[5] Cierny III G. Infected tibial nonunions (1981–1995). The evolution of change. Clin Orthop Relat Res 1999;Mar(360):97–105.

[6] Brinker MR, Bailey Jr DE. Fracture healing in tibia fractures with an associated vascular injury. J Trauma 1997;42:11–9.

[7] Dickson K, Katzman S, Delgado E, et al. Delayed unions and nonunions of open tibial fractures. Correlation with arteriography results. Clin Orthop Relat Res 1994;May(302):189–93.

[8] Dickson KF, Katzman S, Paiement G. The importance of the blood supply in the healing of tibial fractures. Contemp Orthop 1995;30:489–93.

[9] Raikin SM, Landsman JC, Alexander VA, et al. Effect of nicotine on the rate and strength of long bone fracture healing. Clin Orthop Relat Res 1998;Aug(353):231–7.

[10] Schmitz MA, Finnegan M, Natarajan R, et al. Effect of smoking on tibial shaft fracture healing. Clin Orthop Relat Res 1999;Aug(365):184–200.

[11] Mayr E, Frankel V, Ruter A. Ultrasound—an alternative healing method for nonunions? Arch Orthop Trauma Surg 2000;120:1–8.

[12] Nepola JV, Seabold JE, Marsh JL, et al. Diagnosis of infection in ununited fractures. Combined imaging with indium-111-labeled leukocytes and technetium-99m methylene diphosphonate. J Bone Joint Surg Am 1993;75:1816–22.

[13] Spangehl MJ, Younger AS, Masri BA, et al. Diagnosis of infection following total hip arthroplasty. Instr Course Lect 1998;47:285–95.

[14] Court-Brown CM, Keating JF, Christie J, et al. Exchange intramedullary nailing. Its use in aseptic tibial nonunion. J Bone Joint Surg Br 1995;77:407–11.

[15] Court-Brown CM, McQueen MM. High success rate with exchange nailing to treat tibial shaft aseptic nonunion. J Orthop Trauma 1999;13:274.

[16] Sarmiento A, Latta LL. Functional fracture bracing. J Am Acad Orthop Surg 1999;7(1):66–75.

[17] Hannouche D, Petite H, Sedel L. Current trends in the enhancement of fracture healing. J Bone Joint Surg Br 2001;83:157–64.

[18] Bassett CA, Pawluk RJ, Pilla AA. Acceleration of fracture repair by electromagnetic fields. A surgically noninvasive method. Ann N Y Acad Sci 1974;238:242–62.

[19] Ito H, Shirai Y. The efficacy of ununited tibial fracture treatment using pulsing electromagnetic fields: relation to biological activity on nonunion bone ends. J Nippon Med Sch 2001;68:149–53.

[20] Biedermann R, Martin A, Handle G, et al. Extracorporeal shock waves in the treatment of nonunions. J Trauma 2003;54:936–42.

[21] Goulet JA, Templeman D. Delayed union and nonunion of tibial shaft fractures. Instr Course Lect 1997;46:281–91.

[22] Simon JP, Stuyck J, Hoogmartens M, et al. Posterolateral bone grafting for nonunion of the tibia. Acta Orthop Belg 1992;58:308–13.

[23] Rijnberg WJ, van Linge B. Central grafting for persistent nonunion of the tibia. A lateral approach to the tibia, creating a central compartment. J Bone Joint Surg Br 1993;75:926–31.

[24] Ueng SW, Chuang DC, Cheng SL, et al. Management of large infected tibial defects with radical debridement and staged double-rib composite free transfer. J Trauma 1996;40:345–50.

[25] Ueng SW, Wei FC, Shih CH. Management of large infected tibial defects with antibiotic beads local therapy and staged fibular osteoseptocutaneous free transfer. J Trauma 1997;43: 268–74.

[26] DeOrio JK, Ware AW. Salvage technique for treatment of periplafond tibial fractures: the modified fibula-pro-tibia procedure. Foot Ankle Int 2003;24:228–32.

[27] Garg NK, Gaur S, Sharma S. Percutaneous autogenous bone marrow grafting in 20 cases of ununited fracture. Acta Orthop Scand 1993;64:671–2.

[28] Hernigou P, Poignard A, Beaujean F, et al. Percutaneous autologous bone-marrow grafting for nonunions. Influence of the number and concentration of progenitor cells. J Bone Joint Surg Am 2005;87:1430–7.

[29] Urist MR. Bone: transplants, implants, derivatives, and substitutes—a survey of research of the past decade. Instr Course Lect 1960;17:184–95.

[30] Friedlaender GE, Perry CR, Cole JD, et al. Osteogenic protein-1 (bone morphogenetic protein-7) in the treatment of tibial nonunions. J Bone Joint Surg Am 2001;83-A(Suppl 1):S151–8.

[31] Govender S, Csimma C, Genant HK, et al. Recombinant human bone morphogenetic protein-2 for treatment of open tibial fractures: a prospective, controlled, randomized study of four hundred and fifty patients. J Bone Joint Surg Am 2002;84-A:2123–34.

[32] Furlong AJ, Giannoudis PV, DeBoer P, et al. Exchange nailing for femoral shaft aseptic nonunion. Injury 1999;30:245–9.

[33] Wu CC, Shih CH, Chen WJ, et al. High success rate with exchange nailing to treat a tibial shaft aseptic nonunion. J Orthop Trauma 1999;13:33–8.

[34] Mercado EM, Lim EV, Stern PJ, et al. Exchange nailing for failure of initially rodded tibial shaft fractures. Orthopedics 2001;24:757–62.

[35] Templeman D, Thomas M, Varecka T, et al. Exchange reamed intramedullary nailing for delayed union and nonunion of the tibia. Clin Orthop Relat Res 1995;Jun(315):169–75.

[36] Wiss DA, Johnson DL, Miao M. Compression plating for non-union after failed external fixation of open tibial fractures. J Bone Joint Surg Am 1992;74:1279–85.

[37] Helfet DL, Jupiter JB, Gasser S. Indirect reduction and tension-band plating of tibial non-union with deformity. J Bone Joint Surg Am 1992;74:1286–97.

[38] Blatter G, Weber BG. Wave plate osteosynthesis as a salvage procedure. Arch Orthop Trauma Surg 1990;109:330–3.

[39] Karnezis IA. Biomechanical considerations in 'biological' femoral osteosynthesis: an experimental study of the 'bridging' and 'wave' plating techniques. Arch Orthop Trauma Surg 2000; 120:272–5.

[40] Chin KR, Nagarkatti DG, Miranda MA, et al. Salvage of distal tibia metaphyseal nonunions with the 90 degrees cannulated blade plate. Clin Orthop Relat Res 2003;Apr(409):241–9.

[41] Harvey EJ, Henley MB, Swiontkowski MF, et al. The use of a locking custom contoured blade plate for peri-articular nonunions. Injury 2003;34:111–6.

[42] Reed LK, Mormino MA. Functional outcome after blade plate reconstruction of distal tibia metaphyseal nonunions: a study of 11 cases. J Orthop Trauma 2004;18:81–6.

[43] Kabata T, Tsuchiya H, Sakurakichi K, et al. Reconstruction with distraction osteogenesis for juxta-articular nonunions with bone loss. J Trauma 2005;58:1213–22.

[44] Jain AK, Sinha S. Infected nonunion of the long bones. Clin Orthop Relat Res 2005;Feb(431): 57–65.

[45] Brinker RM. Nonunion and malunion. Philadelphia: Saunders; 2003.

[46] Friedrich B, Klaue P. Mechanical stability and post-traumatic osteitis: an experimental evaluation of the relation between infection of bone and internal fixation. Injury 1977;9:23–9.

[47] Schwartsman V, Choi SH, Schwartsman R. Tibial nonunions. Treatment tactics with the Ilizarov method. Orthop Clin North Am 1990;21:639–53.

[48] Cierny III G, Mader JT, Penninck JJ. A clinical staging system for adult osteomyelitis. Clin Orthop Relat Res 2003;Sep(414):7–24.

[49] Venturi ML, Attinger CE, Mesbahi AN, et al. Mechanisms and clinical applications of the vacuum-assisted closure (VAC) device: a review. Am J Clin Dermatol 2005;6:185–94.

[50] Ostermann PA, Seligson D, Henry SL. Local antibiotic therapy for severe open fractures. A review of 1085 consecutive cases. J Bone Joint Surg Br 1995;77:93–7.

[51] McKee MD, Wild LM, Schemitsch EH, et al. The use of an antibiotic-impregnated, osteoconductive, bioabsorbable bone substitute in the treatment of infected long bone defects: early results of a prospective trial. J Orthop Trauma 2002;16:622–7.

[52] Yajima H, Kobata Y, Shigematsu K, et al. Vascularized fibular grafting in the treatment of methicillin-resistant *Staphylococcus aureus* osteomyelitis and infected nonunion. J Reconstr Microsurg 2004;20:13–20.

[53] Amr SM, El-Mofty AO, Amin SN. Anterior versus posterior approach in reconstruction of infected nonunion of the tibia using the vascularized fibular graft: potentialities and limitations. Microsurgery 2002;22:91–107.

ELSEVIER
SAUNDERS

Foot Ankle Clin N Am
11 (2006) 19–33

FOOT AND
ANKLE CLINICS

Tibial Malunion

Anthony P. Mechrefe, MD, Eugene Y. Koh, MD, PhD,
Peter G. Trafton, MD, Christopher W. DiGiovanni, MD*

*Department of Orthopaedic Surgery, Brown Medical School, Rhode Island Hospital,
1287 North Main Street, Providence, RI 02903, USA*

Treatment goals for tibial fractures include timely healing, restoration of normal anatomy, and functional rehabilitation. Deformity that develops during this healing process results in malunion. Malalignment may or may not affect the outcome of a patient who has a tibial shaft fracture. Visible deformity may be well tolerated, even if unsightly, although for some patients malalignment is associated with pain or impaired function and may cause arthritis of the ankle or knee. A surgeon is often consulted after tibial fracture because of (1) pain in the foot, ankle, or knee; (2) a disturbed gait; or (3) apparent or perceived deformity. Pain at the fracture site is more likely to be the result of an occult nonunion rather than from the misalignment itself. Clinical assessment should characterize the patient's complaints, define the patient's deformity by assessing the alignment of both lower extremities, and decide if the pain and impaired function are due to the deformity. Other pathology-causing symptoms, such as ankle arthritis, should also be assessed. The surgeon is obligated to try to establish if the deformity is likely to lead to future problems if left uncorrected but unfortunately there is still no definitive test for determining the degree of misalignment that causes symptoms, nor whether correction will avoid future problems. The decision to correct malunion requires the surgeon's clinical judgment. If the deformity is contributing to symptoms the options for correction should be considered and discussed with the patient. Elective correction of a malunion by a surgeon who is experienced in treating tibial fracture malunions usually is successful, although many potential errors and complications can compromise outcome. Consultation is appropriate for cases that require unfamiliar types of treatment and that have associated risk factors that affect bone or soft tissue healing. The planned

* Corresponding author.
E-mail address: yodigi@aol.com (C.W. DiGiovanni).

1083-7515/06/$ – see front matter © 2006 Elsevier Inc. All rights reserved.
doi:10.1016/j.fcl.2005.12.004

correction may not entirely restore the lower extremity alignment, and it is impossible to know how a given patient will tolerate deformity after healing. Therefore, prevention of malunion is an important part of the acute care of tibial fractures. With well-executed initial treatment and careful follow-up during fracture healing, malunion can be rendered infrequent. Usually, it is easier to prevent deformity rather than to correct it, and easier to correct malalignment in a healing fracture rather than after it has united.

Definition and natural history

A malunited tibial fracture has healed in a clinically unacceptable position. Deformity—significant deviation from normal anatomic configuration—often can be assessed best by comparison with the opposite lower extremity, if it is not itself abnormal. Several factors contribute to deformity [1–12]. The deformity may be any combination of translation and rotation in three planes. The site of a deformity has an affect on outcome and ease of surgical treatment. The fractures may be isolated or multilevel, as might occur with a segmentally comminuted fracture. Angular alignment is assessed with anteroposterior (AP) and lateral radiographs, by two orthogonal views that infer three-dimensional anatomy. When angulation is seen on both views then angular deformity exists in a single plane that is oblique to the sagittal and coronal planes. Fluoroscopic scanning can determine the true plane of deformity by assessing the rotation in which the deformity is most apparent and least visible. Rotational and translational deformity often coexist.

A critical threshold of deformity for predicting symptoms or the potential for arthritis of the ankle and knee has not been outlined. Proximal tibial deformities are likely to affect the knee, whereas distal ones are likely to affect the ankle. Leg length inequality may be associated with low back pain and abnormal gait [2,4,8]. The foot and ankle surgeon may discover that a malunited tibia is the cause of a patient's foot pain as a result of plantar overload. This can be along the lateral column in the event of excessive varus, or within the sinus tarsi or subfibular region with extreme valgus. Varus tibial deformity is less well tolerated because subtalar joint motion may be insufficient to permit a plantigrade foot during stance [1,8,13,14]. Chronic tibial malalignment may lead to progressive degenerative changes of the knee and ankle by eccentrically loading the joints and increasing joint contact pressures in a nonanatomic pattern. The ability of joints to tolerate deformity depends on the amount of preexisting osteoarthritis, the degree of joint injury, the degree and location of fracture deformity, the soft tissue injury, and the presence of infection locally. Patient factors, such as age and comorbidities, have a major affect on healing potential and outcome. Kettelkamp and colleagues [2] investigated degenerative arthritis of the knee after tibial and femoral malunions in a retrospective review of 14 patients with an average follow-up of 31.7 years. Increased force on the medial or lateral tibial plateau that is due to malunion may cause varus or valgus arthritis, respectively, at the knee. Patients who have a minor angular deformity may develop arthritis, and the investigators believed that every effort should be made to obtain an anatomic alignment. van der Schoot and colleagues [12] followed 88 patients after tibial fractures for a mean follow-up of 15 years; 49% had healed with malalignment of at least 5°. They found a statistically significant ($P<.001$) relationship between tibial malalignment and arthritis of the knee and ankle compared with the joints of the contralateral, uninjured side. Puno and colleagues [8] found that the level of eventual dysfunction paralleled the level of deformity. Twenty-seven patients with 28 tibial shaft fractures were evaluated at an average of 8.2 years after their injury. They demonstrated more severe clinical results in the face of greater degrees of ankle malalignment, and statistically significantly higher percentages of good and excellent results with less malalignment.

Other investigators have not confirmed a relationship between tibial malalignment after fracture and degenerative arthritis. Merchant and Dietz [5] evaluated 37 patients who had tibial shaft fractures at an average of 29 years after injury. All of their patients were treated with plaster casts, and had uncomplicated healing of their fractures. Clinical assessment revealed good to excellent results in 78% of ankles and 92% of knees. Radiographic assessment revealed good or excellent results in 76% of ankles and an excellent result for 92% of the knees. They found no correlation between angulation, fracture site, and outcome at the knee or ankle joints. Milner and colleagues [6] investigated the long-term outcome of tibial shaft fractures in 164 patients 30 to 43 years after injury. They evaluated the effect of fracture malunion on the rate of disability, clinical and radiographic signs of arthritis, and self-reported joint pain or stiffness. There was no significant association with malunion angulation of more than 10°, rotation malunion of more than 20°, or shortening of more than 2 cm. Kristensen and colleagues [15] reviewed the rate of restricted motion, pain, and ankle arthrosis 20 to 39 years after injury in 92 patients who were treated nonoperatively for tibial shaft fractures. There was no restriction of motion in 15 patients who had more than 10° of angulation. None of the 22 patients who had angular malunions had radiographic evidence of knee or ankle arthritis. They concluded that angular deformity with 15° can be tolerated without significant risk of ankle arthritis.

Experimental work with rabbits showed arthritic changes after osteotomy, depending on the time of follow-up. Lovasz and colleagues [16] produced 30° varus and valgus osteotomies of the tibia in rabbits and assessed them at 12 weeks. They found only mild articular cartilage changes on histologic, scanning electron microscopic, and immunohistochemical evaluation. Wu and colleagues [17] did a similar experiment, but with longer follow-up (34 weeks). Gross specimen, radiographic, and histochemical evaluation of the specimens revealed severe articular changes, including osteophytes, derangement of cell columns, cloning, fibrillation, and an increase in subchondral bone density.

There is a complex relationship between tibial fracture malunion and poor outcome. A symptomatic patient may be improved by correction of the deformity. Although arthritis may result from unbalanced, repetitive loading of a poorly aligned knee or ankle, there is no consensus about the limit of deformity resulting in arthritis. The decision to recommend surgical correction is based on three factors: symptom severity, functional deficit, and degree of deformity. Generally, patients can tolerate angulation of 5° to 8°, malrotation of up to 15° to 20°, and shortening of 2 cm. Although the surgeon should strive for anatomic alignment during fracture care and as a goal after corrective osteotomy, it is rare for a patient to have significant symptoms that are due to deformity within these limits.

Assessment of the patient

When evaluating a patient with complaints after a tibial fracture, the surgeon must consider more than the patient's chief complaint. A thorough history may localize pain to more than one site. The duration and possible progression of pain and its relationship to activity, severity, and measures that make it better or worse are determined. Other sites of pain (eg, the back) may coexist. Treatment may include a partially completed rehabilitation program or medication. The symptoms may be improving, may have plateaued, or may be deteriorating. The physician should inquire about the patient's perception of deformity and awareness of it. Physical examination should include observation of stance, gait, visible deformity, range of motion, stability (of joints and of fracture site), strength, and tenderness. The deformity may be visible. Leg-length discrepancy should be measured by blocks and a tape measurement from the hip to ankle. The foot may be in external rotation during gait. Rotational alignment with respect to the femur and tibial tubercle as well as the degree of equinus deformity should be assessed. The subtalar joint motion should accommodate for any varus or valgus deformity in the distal tibia. The deformity can overload the medial or lateral border of the foot and cause callus formation. The quality of soft tissue and skin coverage throughout the lower extremity is assessed. A neurovascular assessment completes the examination.

Radiographs should include a full AP, lateral, and both oblique views of the tibia. Healing, tibial bone structure, and the knee and ankle joints are assessed. It is necessary to determine the presence, location, and severity of deformity [3,7,18,19]. Paley's methodology is effective to analyze and correct skeletal deformity [20,21]. An AP standing radiograph with the patient bearing weight on both legs is mandatory for proper assessment. The camera is 10 feet from the patient and centered on the knee joint. The film cassette must be long enough to include both lower extremities, from hip to ankle joints. Both patellae should point forward and be centered over their knee joints to control rotation. The centers of the hip, knee, and ankle joints are outlined. The AP mechanical axis is a line that connects the center of the femoral head to the center of the ankle joint. The mechanical axis deviation (MAD) is the distance from the center of the knee to the mechanical axis, perpendicular to the mechanical axis. The normal MAD averages 8 ± 7 mm medial to the mechanical axis. It is compared with the MAD of the opposite leg, because patient variability is considerable. The MAD can be estimated in the operating room from a fluoroscopic view of the knee using the electrocautery wire tensioned from the center of the femoral head to the center of the ankle joint. This test is sensitive for frontal plane deformity near the knee.

To assess deformity near the ankle, the tibial anatomic axis is drawn on a film taken with the foot perpendicular to the film cassette, parallel to the central ray. If there is tibial deformity, the axis of the distal segment—rather than the entire tibia—should be used. This axis line, which represents the tibial shaft (or distal segment) is drawn to cross the ankle joint line. The angle on the lateral side between the ankle joint line and the distal part of the tibial anatomic axis (lateral distal tibial angle, normally $89° \pm 3°$) is measured and compared with the opposite side. This establishes the alignment of the ankle joint with the shaft on the AP view. Similar joint line–shaft alignment measurements are done at the knee on AP and lateral views (medial proximal tibial angle, $87.5° \pm 2.5°$; anatomic proximal posterior tibial angle, $81° \pm 4°$) and at the ankle in the lateral view to calculate the anatomic anterior distal tibial angle ($5° \pm 2°$). Typically, the knee joint line on the lateral view is intersected by the tibial shaft axis in the anterior one fifth of the joint. The lateral ankle joint line is bisected by the tibial anatomic axis. Sagittal plane limb alignment is measured by using the mechanical axis on a long-leg view; however, rotation in the presence of knee flexion or contracture causes errors in measurement. It is easier to approximate sagittal plane alignment with a "pick-up test" showing a straight lower limb when lifted off the operating room table (maximal gravity knee extension), with neither apex–anterior nor apex–posterior angulation.

Angular deformity can be measured from the anatomic axis of each tibial segment. The anatomic axis is a line joining two midline diaphyseal points bisecting the transverse diameter of the tibia proximally and distally in each segment. The line from the proximal segment is extended until it crosses the distal segment. Paley [20] called the junction the "center of rotation of angulation" (CORA). The angle between the axes of proximal and distal segments is the angle of deformity. Correction reduces this angle to $0°$. Typically, the CORA coincides with the obvious apex of deformity. This is not be the case with occasion translational deformity or when there is more than one level of deformity. Periarticular alignment is hard to measure. The anatomic axis is harder to determine in the metaphyseal region; the appropriate segmental axis is determined better by drawing the joint line and using the normal angles to draw the axis line on AP and lateral views at appropriate angles from the midpoint of the AP knee and ankle joint lines.

Typically, displacement is seen on AP and lateral radiographs, because it is in a different plane to the radiographic views. Paley [20] showed how this can be measured graphically by plotting the AP displacement on the horizontal axis, and the lateral displacement on the vertical axis. Perpendiculars to these points meet and form a rectangle. Starting at the graph's origin, a diagonal line is drawn to the far corner of this rectangle. Its length, adjusting to the scale of the radiographs, is that of the displacement, and the angle between that line and the axes reflects the true direction of displacement. The amount of displacement that must be corrected also is indicated by the distance that remains between the segmental axes after angulation is corrected to make them parallel.

Leg-length discrepancy can be measured using calibrated blocks, long-leg scanograms, or with a ruler positioned from hip to ankle. The CT imaging scanograms are most accurate. Positioning the patient prone and flexing the knee 90° can establish whether the leg-length discrepancy is in the tibial or femoral segment [18].

Tibial rotation can be assessed by measuring the thigh–foot angle, with the knee flexed 90° [18]. This also can be measured by using CT cuts through the proximal and distal tibia. The angle between the ankle's intermalleolar line and one tangent to the posterior proximal tibial condyles should be similar bilaterally. The difference between the normal side and the abnormal side indicates the angle of malrotation.

Treatment options

Patients should exhaust nonoperative measures, including shoe modifications or bracing. Other measures include anti-inflammatory or analgesic medication, activity modification, and orthoses. Medial or lateral off-loading braces for the knee, ankle–foot orthoses for the ankle, and orthotic wear or shoe lifts for the foot may accommodate deformities that produce mild to moderate symptoms. Ambulatory aids, such as canes, crutches, or walkers, can provide additional benefit. If the patient does not have a plantigrade foot or a functional limb position or has malaligned knee and ankle joints with asymmetric loading, treatment weighs in favor of corrective osteotomy. This might be more advisable if the patient has symptomatic osteoarthritis or radiographic evidence of unilateral excessive joint loading. If the patient is comfortable, reassessment every 6 months is preferable.

When nonoperative treatment fails surgical treatment should be considered. The alternatives include immediate correction by way of osteotomy and fixation; progressive correction with osteotomy and external fixation; and salvage surgery; including arthroplasty or fusion, perhaps with the addition of osteotomy for deformity correction. Amputation also should be considered and discussed, particularly in the case of severe deformity with local or systemic comorbidities.

Planning deformity correction

After the tibial deformity has been analyzed as described above, a plan for its correction can be developed [1,3,7,11,18,19,22]. Paley's [20] text describes this in meticulous detail. The reader is referred to this text for a comprehensive, well-illustrated discussion.

A full-scale tracing of the patient's normal tibia can provide a template for the desired correction.. Tracings of the proximal and distal segments of the malaligned tibia are superimposed on the AP and lateral views. The effects of different types of osteotomies can be compared, and one can be selected. The osteotomy should be at the level of the CORA.

Depending upon the axis around which the distal segment is rotated to achieve correction, an opening or closing wedge might be created. Any points on a line that bisects the transverse angle at the CORA can be used as centers of rotation for angular correction. If the osteotomy is at a different level from the CORA, translation of the axes occurs, unless the axis for the correction of angulation is at the CORA of the deformity. This may assist in deformity correction if a translational deformity is also present. Several different osteotomy locations and configurations might be considered. Risks and benefits of each should be considered. Other factors include the healing potential of the bone at the level of the osteotomy, and the need for a fibular osteotomy. Bone grafting should be considered. Salvage of a wound slough, infection, or nonunion should be considered before surgery.

The soft tissue envelope at the level of a potential osteotomy should be assessed. This may affect the incision used, the fixation chosen, and the wound healing. Hardware should be placed away from any at-risk wounds or incisions. When large degrees of correction are performed adjacent neurovascular structures may be stretched detrimentally by corrective osteotomies or lengthening procedures [11,19]. For example, correction of significant valgus deformity in the proximal tibia may injure the common peroneal nerve. In these rare cases, particularly if there is shortening or poor soft tissue, consideration should be given to osteotomy and gradual deformity correction using distraction osteogenesis with external fixation, as described by Ilizarov [7,11,20,21].

The fixation technique that is chosen to perform correction is based upon the degree of deformity, the presence of a limb-length discrepancy, the condition of the soft tissue envelope, and the experience of the surgeon. Numerous methods have been described, including oblique osteotomy with lag screw and neutralization plate fixation; opening, closing, or neutral wedge osteotomy; dome osteotomy; intramedullary nailing; and external fixation devices with distraction histogenesis.

A complete assessment and treatment planning must be individualized. Several solutions may be possible. Ultimately, the surgeon and patient can choose the one that is best for the patient and surgical team. Certain principles must be observed. Osteotomies are performed atraumatically, by avoiding excessive soft tissue stripping, to maximize healing potential. Osteotomies should be done slowly, with a cooled saw, to avoid thermal injury of the bone. Correction with rotational osteotomies or closing wedges are preferable to opening ones to decrease the risks of wound tension and to minimize the requirements for bone grafting. Strict attention should be paid to planning access through the soft tissue envelope for osteotomy and fixation. The soft tissues must be healthy enough to permit some stretch during correction and to permit tension-free coverage over hardware and bone graft. Gentle retraction minimizes healing complications. Postoperative compartment syndrome can occur. Contractures of nearby joints are common in patients who have tibial deformity, particularly when the problem is long-standing. They can impact outcome if not addressed concomitantly with correction of osseous deformity. Often, this is performed best with percutaneous techniques in the event of Achilles (equinus) contracture; however, occasionally it necessitates formal open arthrotomy and release of the ankle or knee which must be considered in the context of the other necessary exposures before surgery is performed.

Inexperienced surgeons may wish to consult a specialist who is familiar with the planning and execution of tibial osteotomies for posttraumatic deformity, particularly for complicated deformities or corrections. Operating with a more experienced colleague improves the safety and ease of these procedures, which are performed rarely.

Osteotomy

Osteotomy location must be planned carefully. It should allow for correction of deformity as discussed above, but also should be placed in a site with good healing potential. Diaphyseal osteotomies tend to heal slowly. Percutaneous procedures with multiple drill holes, minimal soft tissue stripping, and intramedullary fixation may counteract this, as may exposure through decortication using an osteotome to produce multiple, thin cortical fragments that remain vascularized through their attachments to surrounding soft tissues [11,20,21,23]. Metaphyseal osteotomies tend to heal more reliably, but must be placed to permit correction of deformity, and to have as much bone contact area as possible while preserving sufficient bone stock in the articular fragment for adequate fixation. Valuable osteotomies include oblique metaphyseal osteotomies and focal dome osteotomies [23]. When a nailed tibial fracture has healed with malrotation, a metadiaphyseal Afghan osteotomy [24]—after removal of the initial nail—allows correction of moderate deformity, and can be fixed with another locked tibial nail. Usually, fibular osteotomy is required.

Fixation

For metaphyseal osteotomies, fixation with absolute stability is necessary. This may include lag screws and neutralization plates or compression plating with a fixed angle device (blade-plate or plate with locked screws) that provides optimal purchase in the short articular bone segment. The osteotomy is compressed using an external tension device. Intramedullary nails rarely are a good choice for fixing a proximal or distal tibial osteotomy. An associated fibular osteotomy should be transfixed for additional stability. For a diaphyseal osteotomy with an open medullary canal that can be aligned congruently, intramedullary fixation should be considered because of its durability, possibility for earlier weight bearing, and potential avoidance of extensive exposure. If extensive exposure is required to correct deformity, the surgeon should approach the bone with decortication rather than subperiosteal dissection, and bone grafting should be considered.

Intramedullary nailing can be used for fixation for diaphyseal osteotomies [17,25,26]. Contraindications to intramedullary nailing are lack of a coaxial medullary canal and not having long enough segments for adequate fixation. Previous infection also is a relative contraindication. In a series of 24 malunions that was treated with intramedullary fixation, union was achieved in 22 (95%) of the patients [25]. Another series of 14 malunions and nonunions that was

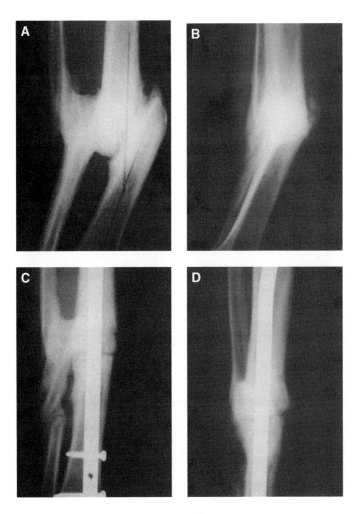

Fig. 1. (A) AP radiograph of midshaft tibia malunion in a 32-year-old man that was treated with a long leg cast and functional cast bracing. (B) Oblique radiograph of tibial malunion. (C) AP radiograph of tibia after osteotomy and intramedullary nailing of the tibia fracture. (D) Lateral radiograph of healed corrected tibial malunion.

treated with intramedullary nailing achieved similar results, with union in 13 (93%) patients [26]. Wu and colleagues [17] described 37 consecutive tibial malunions that were treated with intramedullary nailing. All patients had a fibulotomy, closing wedge osteotomy, cancellous bone grafting, and open reaming of the medullary canal. Thirty-four patients were followed for an average of 1 year; all had achieved union and demonstrated full range of motion of the knee and ankle, preoperatively and postoperatively. Generally, these devices should be locked statically for maximal stability and maintenance of alignment (Fig. 1).

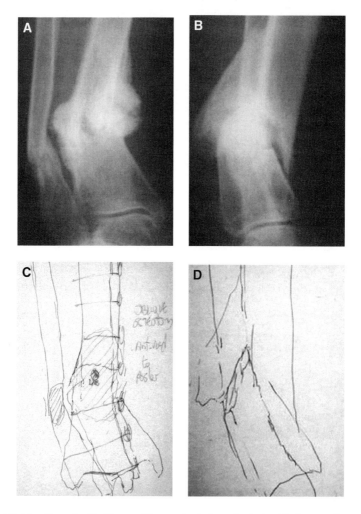

Fig. 2. (*A*) AP radiograph of a 25-year-old man who had a malunited ankle fracture after treatment in a fiberglass cast. (*B*) Lateral radiograph of ankle showing angular deformity. (*C, D*) Preoperative plan showing tracings of planned osteotomy and fixation. (*E*) Intraoperative radiograph of reduction. (*F*) Patient 1 year after corrective osteotomy with restored alignment.

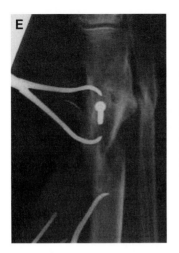
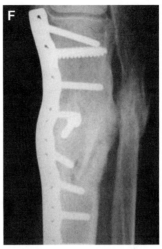

Fig. 2 (*continued*).

An oblique, properly oriented osteotomy is well suited to correction of complex metadiaphyseal deformities. Any angular deformity can be corrected with a single appropriate cut [27]. The osteotomy's broad surface helps to gain stable fixation and good bone contact for healing. Transverse plane displacement can be corrected to an extent, as can shortening, by shearing the osteotomy in the desired direction. Fixation is done with a lag screw and neutralization plate. Intraoperative fluoroscopy is used to obtain the true plane of the deformity [19]. Two 6.0-mm Schanz pins, which are placed proximally and distally parallel to the joint surfaces of the knee and ankle, respectively, are connected with a femoral distractor (Synthes USA, Paoli, Pennsylvania). A single oblique osteotomy is made perpendicular to the plane of the deformity, and the correction is obtained using the distractor and pointed reduction clamps. A lag screw is placed across the osteotomy after the length is adjusted, and alignment is corrected. Full AP and lateral tibial radiographs confirm alignment. A neutralization plate is placed to protect stability. In Sanders and colleagues' [19] series of 15 patients, the average preoperative coronal plane deformity measured 14°, the average sagittal plane deformity measured 13°, and the average leg-length discrepancy was 2.2 cm. The mean follow up was 25 months. At the latest follow-up, 10 patients had an excellent result. The average correction in the coronal plane was within 1° of normal, the average correction in the sagittal plane was within 2° of normal, and the average lengthening was 1.3 cm. Care must be undertaken when performing oblique osteotomies because they may introduce deformity in other planes, including malrotation. Wedge-shaped segments from the osteotomy site are used to achieve proper reduction. These segments can be used for later bone grafting (Fig. 2).

Metaphyseal dome osteotomies are best suited to correct metaphyseal deformity without the need for length adjustment. Because some osteotomies are based on the CORA it does not result in axis shift, and its good bone contact promotes rapid healing (Fig. 3).

Traction histogenesis

External fixation is a means of stabilizing osteotomies and achieving correction of malunited bones. An external fixation device is preferable in the setting

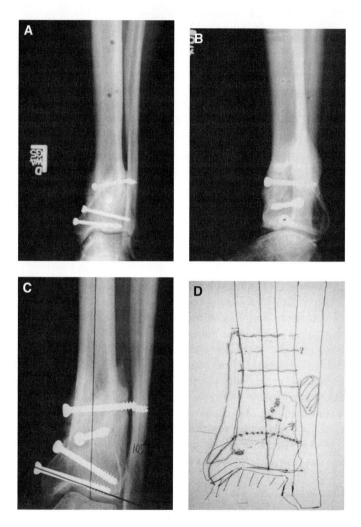

Fig. 3. (*A*) AP radiograph of a 42-year-old woman who had a malunion after open reduction and internal fixation of an open distal tibia fracture. (*B*) Lateral radiograph of malunited fracture. (*C*) AP radiograph of ankle. (*D*) Preoperative plan showing tracings of dome osteotomy and plate fixation. (*E*) AP radiograph of healed osteotomy. (*F*) Lateral radiograph after corrective osteotomy.

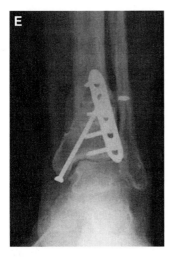
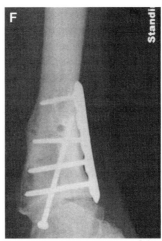

Fig. 3 (*continued*).

of infection; poor soft tissue envelopes that are not amenable to large exposures; limb length discrepancy; or multilevel, multiplanar deformity. Paley and
colleagues [7] have extensive experience using an Ilizarov-type external fixator
to achieve correction. The circular Ilizarov-type frame provides six degrees of
freedom in correction, and multiple rings can be placed to correct multilevel deformities. The Ilizarov frame is rigid enough to provide the stability necessary to
support regenerate bone during deformity correction and bone consolidation.
Paley and colleagues [7] reported using the Ilizarov technique in 22 tibial
malunions. All patients had lengthening and had complete elimination of angular
rotation and translational deformity when the fixator was removed. More
recently, Feldman and colleagues [22] described their experience with the Taylor
spatial frame (TSF; Smith & Nephew, Memphis, Tennessee), which provides
similar versatility with the added advantage of a computer program to guide
correction. In their series of 18 patients who had tibial malunions and nonunions
that were treated with the TSF, 17 patients achieved union and significant correction of their deformities in six axes (coronal angulation and translation, sagittal
angulation and translation, rotation, and shortening). The mean residual angular
deformity was 1.8°, the mean residual translational deformity was 1.3 mm, and
all rotational deformities were corrected. Fifteen of 17 (88%) patients returned
to their preinjury activities.

Complications

The major complications of malunion surgery, regardless of technique, include
failure to achieve or maintain correction, wound slough, neurovascular injury,
nonunion, and infection. To prevent complications the surgeon must identify

the goals and requirements of surgical correction and must have the right equipment. Patient factors may complicate any attempt at correction, before entertaining these procedures. Surgical time must be minimized by good preoperative planning, gentle surgical technique, and careful postoperative follow-up. Postoperative noncompliance and neuropathic patients can affect outcome adversely.

Results

Results of malunion surgery indicate that the surgical expertise that is required increases with the complexity of the malunion. To achieve good outcomes, multiplanar, multilevel deformities that require osteotomy and progressive deformity correction with distraction histogenesis should be reserved for surgeons who specialize in this surgery. Long-term results after malunion surgery depend upon numerous factors, including preexisting arthrosis of the knee and ankle, ipsilateral hindfoot and midfoot pathology, joint contractures, and the condition of the overlying soft tissues.

Summary

Tibial malunions are prevented best by careful management of acute fractures, with appropriate intervention to correct developing deformity. Indications for surgical intervention include patients who have symptoms and deformity, and those who are asymptomatic but who have significant deformity that may cause progressive posttraumatic arthrosis. Surgical planning includes thorough patient education, creation of realistic expectations, assessment of risk/benefit ratios, accurate definition of deformity, and careful selection of implants and approach. There is no universal algorithm for determining the amount of deformity that requires osteotomy, and which type is best for a given patient. Treatment should be individualized based on the deformity, an appropriate assessment of risks and benefits, and the potential for wound complications. Observing a patient over time may provide insight into the need for surgery. Documentation of symptom progression can clarify the need for surgery. Given the variety of surgical options and the relative rarity of osteotomies for tibial malunion, a second opinion may be helpful before surgery is performed.

References

[1] Johnson KD. Management of malunion and nonunion of the tibia. Orthop Clin North Am 1987; 18(1):157–71.
[2] Kettelkamp DB, Hillberry BM, Murrish DE, et al. Degenerative arthritis of the knee secondary to fracture malunion. Clin Orthop Relat Res 1988;Sep(234):159–69.
[3] Mast JW, Teitge RA, Gowda M. Preoperative planning for the treatment of nonunions and the correction of malunions of the long bones. Orthop Clin North Am 1990;21(4):693–714.

[4] McKellop HA, Llinas A, Sarmiento A. Effects of tibial malalignment on the knee and ankle. Orthop Clin North Am 1994;25(3):415–23.

[5] Merchant TC, Dietz FR. Long-term follow-up after fractures of the tibial and fibular shafts. J Bone Joint Surg Am 1989;71(4):599–606.

[6] Milner SA, Davis TR, Muir KR, et al. Long-term outcome after tibial shaft fracture: is malunion important? J Bone Joint Surg Am 2002;84-A(6):971–80.

[7] Paley D, Chaudray M, Pirone AM, et al. Treatment of malunions and mal-nonunions of the femur and tibia by detailed preoperative planning and the Ilizarov techniques. Orthop Clin North Am 1990;21(4):667–91.

[8] Puno RM, Vaughan JJ, Stetten ML, et al. Long-term effects of tibial angular malunion on the knee and ankle joints. J Orthop Trauma 1991;5(3):247–54.

[9] Shah K, Quaimkhani S. Long-term outcome after tibial shaft fracture: is malunion important? J Bone Joint Surg Am 2004;86-A(2):436 [author reply 436–7].

[10] Tetsworth K, Paley D. Malalignment and degenerative arthropathy. Orthop Clin North Am 1994;25(3):367–77.

[11] Trafton PG. Skeletal trauma: basic science, management, and reconstruction, vol. 2. 3rd edition. Philadelphia: Elsevier; 2003. p. 2131–255.

[12] van der Schoot DK, Den Outer AJ, Bode PJ, et al. Degenerative changes at the knee and ankle related to malunion of tibial fractures. 15-year follow-up of 88 patients. J Bone Joint Surg Br 1996;78(5):722–5.

[13] Olerud C. The effect of the syndesmotic screw on the extension capacity of the ankle joint. Arch Orthop Trauma Surg 1985;104(5):299–302.

[14] Tarr RR, Resnick CT, Wagner KS, et al. Changes in tibiotalar joint contact areas following experimentally induced tibial angular deformities. Clin Orthop Relat Res 1985;Oct(199):72–80.

[15] Kristensen KD, Kiaer T, Blicher J. No arthrosis of the ankle 20 years after malaligned tibial-shaft fracture. Acta Orthop Scand 1989;60(2):208–9.

[16] Lovasz G, Llinas A, Benya P, et al. Effects of valgus tibial angulation on cartilage degeneration in the rabbit knee. J Orthop Res 1995;13(6):846–53.

[17] Wu CC, Chen WJ, Shih CH. Tibial shaft malunion treated with reamed intramedullary nailing: a revised technique. Arch Orthop Trauma Surg 2000;120(3–4):152–6.

[18] Probe RA. Lower extremity angular malunion: evaluation and surgical correction. J Am Acad Orthop Surg 2003;11(5):302–11.

[19] Sanders R, Anglen JO, Mark JB. Oblique osteotomy for the correction of tibial malunion. J Bone Joint Surg Am 1995;77(2):240–6.

[20] Paley D. Principles of deformity correction. Berlin: Springer-Verlag; 2002.

[21] Trafton PG. Tibial shaft fractures. In: Browner BD, Jupiter JB, Levine AM, Trafton PG, editors. Skeletal trauma: basic science, management, and reconstruction, vol. 2. 3rd edition. Philadelphia: Saunders; 2003. p. 2131–255.

[22] Feldman DS, Shin SS, Madan S, et al. Correction of tibial malunion and nonunion with six-axis analysis deformity correction using the Taylor spatial frame. J Orthop Trauma 2003;17(8): 549–54.

[23] Stamatis ED, Myerson MS. Supramalleolar osteotomy: indications and technique. Foot Ankle Clin 2003;8(2):317–33.

[24] Paktiss AS, Gross RH. Afghan percutaneous osteotomy. J Pediatr Orthop 1993;13(4):531–3.

[25] Mayo KA, Benirschke SK. Treatment of tibial malunions and nonunions with reamed intramedullary nails. Orthop Clin North Am 1990;21(4):715–24.

[26] McLaren AC, Blokker CP. Locked intramedullary fixation for metaphyseal malunion and nonunion. Clin Orthop Relat Res 1991;Apr(265):253–60.

[27] Sangeorzan BJ, Sangeorzan BP, Hansen Jr ST, et al. Mathematically directed single-cut osteotomy for correction of tibial malunion. J Orthop Trauma 1989;3(4):267–75.

ELSEVIER
SAUNDERS

Foot Ankle Clin N Am
11 (2006) 35–50

FOOT AND
ANKLE CLINICS

Ankle Syndesmosis Injuries

Fernando A. Peña, MD*, J. Chris Coetzee, MD

*Department of Orthopaedic Surgery, Foot and Ankle Service,
University of Minnesota 2450 Riverside Avenue, Suite R200, Minneapolis, MN 55454, USA*

The incidence of ankle syndesmosis injuries—also known as high ankle sprains—is increasing, in part because of an increased awareness of the diagnosis. The most likely mechanism of injury involves some component of external rotation and eversion; this is different from common lateral ankle sprains that have an inversion internal rotation mechanism of injury. The management of acute and chronic syndesmosis injuries are discussed in this article.

Incidence

The real prevalence of ankle syndesmosis injuries probably is underestimated because many are missed or are not treated acutely. Hopkinson and colleagues [1] suggested that ankle syndesmosis injuries account for 1% of all ankle injuries in the United States military. Fallat and colleagues [2] followed all ankle injuries that presented at a local emergency department and a primary care clinic prospectively for 33 months. The diagnosis of a high syndesmosis injury was made on physical examination without any further investigation. Of 639 patients who had 547 soft tissue injuries and 92 ankle fractures, the prevalence of syndesmosis injuries was 0.5%. In contrast, Boytin and colleagues [3] reported a prevalence of 18% for syndesmosis injuries in a prospective study of 98 ankle injuries. The diagnosis was reached by physical examination. The emphasis of the study was placed on the length of time that it took to recover from a syndesmosis injury compared with a lateral ankle sprain. The high prevalence of ankle syndesmosis injuries in this subpopulation of professional football players

* Corresponding author.
E-mail address: pena0013@umn.edu (F.A. Peña).

1083-7515/06/$ – see front matter © 2006 Elsevier Inc. All rights reserved.
doi:10.1016/j.fcl.2005.12.007
foot.theclinics.com

can be explained easily by the rules and contact that is sustained during the practice of football. That percentage should not be extrapolated to the more standard population. As a rare injury, the diagnosis may be missed and appropriate treatment may be delayed.

Anatomy

The ankle syndesmosis is the joint between the distal tibia and the distal fibula. Motion at this joint includes some translation and rotation during tibiotalar dorsiflexion and plantarflexion to accommodate the asymmetric talus while maintaining congruency [4]. Three main structures provide stability at the syndesmosis: the interosseous tibiofibular ligament, the anterior inferior tibiofibular ligament, and the posterior inferior tibiofibular ligament.

The interosseous tibiofibular ligament represents the distal continuation of the interosseous membrane. At approximately 4 cm to 5 cm above the ankle joint it forms a triangle with a lateral base and a medial apex. Inferiorly, this forms the anterior inferior tibiofibular ligament that is defined from the interosseous ligament by a space. The posterior inferior tibiofibular ligament has a similar relationship. The bulk of the interosseous tibiofibular ligament ends 1 cm to 1.5 cm above the joint line at the upper margin of the three-faceted distal tibiofibular joint.

The anterior inferior tibiofibular ligament forms three fascicles. The middle is the strongest and most prominent. These bundles arise in the vicinity of the anterior distal tibial (Chopart's) tubercle, and insert into the most anterior tubercle of the distal fibula. The superior bundle is proximal to the tubercles, whereas the inferior bundle is distal to the tubercles. The middle bundle travels obliquely from Chaput's tubercle to the distal fibula at a 30° angle to the joint line.

The posterior inferior tibiofibular ligament has less distinct bundles that originate from the posterior tubercle of the tibia and attach into the posterior tubercle of the distal fibula. The direction of the posterior inferior tibiofibular ligament is more horizontal than is the anterior inferior tibiofibular ligament.

The morphology of the distal tibiofibular joint is variable. The distal tibiofibular joint has three facets; the middle is the most consistent. The anterior facet has fibrotic tissue that blends with the anterior inferior fibular ligaments. The variable-sized posterior facet has a plica. This facet is visualized intraarticularly extending proximally into the syndesmosis up to 12 mm to 15 mm from the ankle joint line. The middle facet has a cartilaginous surface that articulates with the lateral tibial facet.

Biomechanics

With ankle dorsiflexion, the distal fibula moves proximally, posteriorly and rotates externally. Beumer and colleagues [5] demonstrated by radiostereometry that an external rotation force rotates the fibula externally and translates it posteromedially.

In a cadaver study, Ogilvie-Harris and colleagues [6] showed that the anterior inferior tibiofibular ligament contributes 35% of the strength of the syndesmosis, the posterior inferior tibiofibular ligament contributes 40%, and the interosseous ligament contributes 21%.

A partial transection of the anterior inferior tibiofibular ligament can provide enough diastases to be clinically significant but not demonstrated by plain radiographic imaging [7]. A translation of 2.3 mm of the talus after complete transaction of the anterior tibiofibular ligament alone will increase to 7.3 mm of translation after complete transaction of all syndesmosis ligaments. Instability may be present, despite having some remaining structures intact.

A missed unstable ankle syndesmosis injury can result in end-stage ankle degeneration; however, the mechanism for degenerative change is not clear. Pereira and colleagues [8] studied the ankle joint kinetics after a complete syndesmosis and deltoid ligament injury. In contrast to other studies, under a full weight-bearing axial load, the talus has a tendency to relocate itself to the most congruent position and restore its symmetry within the mortise, even with a displaced syndesmosis. The likely mechanism for lateral talar shift after syndesmosis injury includes posterior translation of the fibula.

Pathophysiology

An external rotation torque that is applied to the foot may tear the soft tissue structures that are responsible for stability of the ankle syndesmosis; the intraosseous ligament is torn to the knee, a spiral fracture of the fibula may occur low or high (a Maissoneuve fracture), or the intraosseous ligament becomes torn above the fracture site. A high fracture or intraosseous ligament tear may be missed if the proximal leg is not examined.

Clinical presentation and diagnosis

Instability may be the main presenting complaint in an acute ankle syndesmosis injury. In patients who have a chronic injury, pain and functional deficits secondary to a widened syndesmosis are the predominant symptoms.

Acute injuries

The mode of injury indicates the potential for a syndesmosis injury. The patient may have some anterolateral ankle pain proximal to the lateral collateral ligaments. The patient may be able to walk on a straight line, but may have symptoms during external rotation, cutting or shifting directions because of the syndesmosis instability and pain. Swelling or contusion may be minimal.

Physical examination

Special tests have been described to assess a syndesmosis injury. These include the Hopkins (squeeze) test, external rotation under stress test, palpation test, and compression of the syndesmosis with maximum dorsiflexion [9,10]. In a study on the reliability of these tests, the external rotation under stress test was most reliable and the squeeze test, or Hopkins test, was the least valuable. The external rotation test is performed with the knee and ankle at $90°$ and a force with external rotation is applied to the midfoot area. If pain is present, the test is positive. An alternative test that was not studied but that can be performed on less symptomatic patients requires the patient to stand on the affected leg and rotate the pelvis towards the opposite side; this maneuver applies an external rotation torque to the affected ankle which will reproduce pain in the presence of ankle syndesmosis instability.

Diagnostic imaging studies

Standing anteroposterior (AP), lateral, and mortise views should be obtained of both ankles in weight-bearing patients. Patients who have proximal leg tenderness also should have an AP and lateral view of the whole leg. CT scans and MRI scans may be of value in more subtle cases. Examination under anesthesia may be the final test before surgery. On a mortise view a lateral translational force is applied to the ankle; opening of the syndesmosis confirms the diagnosis. A concomitant deltoid ligament injury result in a greater degree of translation [11].

Beumer and colleagues [12] studied motion of the distal fibula before and after a syndesmosis injury in cadavers. The fibula tended to rotate externally after disruption of the syndesmosis. This is hard to visualize on plain radiographs. Posterior translation of the distal fibula on a lateral projection of the ankle joint was seen as a secondary pathology.

Beumer and colleagues [13] concluded in a separate cadaver study that the fibular overlap and the clear space are the most valuable radiographic signs of syndesmosis injury. The clear space is defined as the area created between the lateral cortex of the tibia and the medial one from the fibula at 1 cm above the joint line. A clear space of greater than 6 mm indicates a syndesmosis injury. A widened medial joint space is suggestive of an associated deltoid ligament injury.

In an MRI study, injuries that were associated with a syndesmosis disruption included anterior tibiofibular ligament disruption in 74% of cases, osteochondral lesions of the talus in 28% of cases, and bone bruises in 24% of cases [14]. This study may have overestimated the associated injury rate, but the treating physician should examine for these associated injuries.

Chronic injuries

In the presence of a chronic painful ankle syndesmosis, pain may be due to the presence of scar tissue or the lack of congruency of the syndesmosis and tibiotalar joints. The scar tissue may be present at the level of the syndesmosis or along the medial gutter of the ankle. Scar tissue must be removed to allow reduction of the syndesmosis. A preoperative MRI indicates the size and location of scar tissue.

The congruency of the ankle syndesmosis and the relative position of the fibula with respect to the tibia is assessed best by CT scan. A CT scan can detect 1 mm of syndesmosis displacement, whereas plain radiographs miss 3 mm of displacement 50% of the time [15].

Thordarson and colleagues [16] studied the contact pressures within the ankle joint with any displacement of the fibula in nine fresh frozen cadavers. The fibula was displaced in all three planes, by translation in one single plane as well as a combination of planes, and fixed during the testing sequence with an external fixator. They concluded that shortening was associated with the highest increase in contact pressures, followed by lateral translation of the fibula, or widening of the ankle syndesmosis. A lateral translation of the fibula of 2 mm—the smallest increment that was tested on their experimental sequence—increased the contact pressure by almost 40% from baseline in some of the quadrants on the surface of the talus. Out of all of the quadrants of the talus, the posterolateral one was affected most by the change in position of the fibula (Fig. 1).

Treatment of acute injuries

Takao and colleagues [17] published the results of arthroscopic evaluation of tibiofibular syndesmosis disruption. They collected 38 patients who had Weber B ankle fractures. Using AP and mortise radiography they diagnosed ankle syndesmosis disruption on 42% and 55% of the cases, respectively. With the use of ankle arthroscopy, the diagnosis increased to 87%.

Tornetta and colleagues [18] showed in a cadaver study that overtightening of the intact fibula at the syndesmosis was hard to achieve. It is possible that a fractured fibula may prevent dorsiflexion if the fracture is not anatomic. Therefore, full dorsiflexion of the ankle during screw placement is not required. Instead, attention should be directed at making sure that the fibula is out to length, rotated correctly, and reduced into the syndesmosis with no anterior posterior or lateral translation.

The most reliable way to assess reduction of the syndesmosis is through comparison with the opposite ankle after obtaining an AP, mortise, and lateral

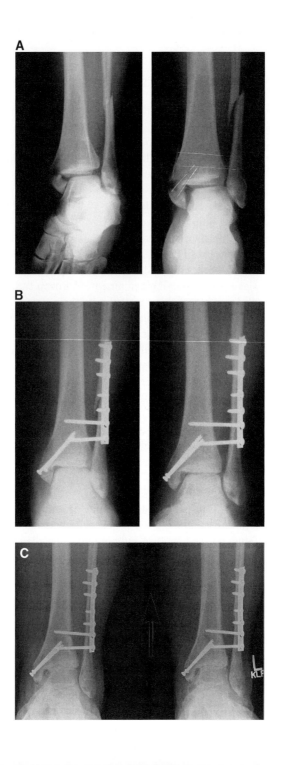

fluoroscopy or radiographic image. The clear space and the overlap of the fibula with the tibia at 1 cm proximal to the joint line are the parameters to analyze on the AP and mortise views. The lateral view helps to assess proper reduction of the fibula with the tibial sulcus. It should have no increased anterior or posterior translation when compared with the noninjured side.

Screw placement, type, and technique

McBryde and colleagues [19] studied the best location for the syndesmosis screw in 17 paired cadaver limbs. A 3.5-mm self-tapping stainless steel cortical screw was used. The specimens were tested to failure through an external rotation torque at 90° per minute. They concluded that a screw which is located 2 cm proximal to the joint line provided better fixation than did one that was 3.5 cm proximal to the joint line (Fig. 2).

Thompson and Gesink [20] studied the biomechanical difference between a 3.5-mm and a 4.5-mm stainless steel screw in cadavers. Three cortices were purchased. The screw pulled out in five out of six specimens that had the 3.5-mm screw, whereas the fibula fractured in five out of the six specimens that had the 4.5-mm screw. The investigators concluded that there was nobiomechanical advantage to using a 4.5-mm tricortical screw for syndesmosis fixation. No washers or plates were used in either group.

Hoiness and Stromsoe [21] followed a randomized group of 64 patients prospectively to evaluate the use of a single tetracortical screw versus two tricortical screws for instability of the syndesmosis. All but three injuries were related to ankle fractures. Although there was no clinical difference between the two groups at 1 year of follow-up, the investigators recommended the use of two tricortical screws because it represented a safe option and improved early function. The number of syndesmosis surgically fixed where there was inherent stability and no need for such fixation, is not clear in clinical studies.

Beumer and colleagues [22] studied the biomechanical behavior of titanium versus stainless steel screws, and the purchasing of three versus four cortices of the ankle syndesmosis on 16 fresh frozen cadavers. Two hundred and twenty-five thousand cycles of axial load were applied through the ankle joint. Despite no fracture of bones or screws, they recorded widening of the syndesmosis of 1.05 mm.

Cox and colleagues [23] studied the biomechanical behavior of 5.0 mm stainless steel screws versus 5.00 mm poly-L-lacticpolyglycolic acid (PLLA-PGA) bioabsorbable screws. Eight paired cadaver limbs were used. A cycling

Fig. 1. (A) Radiographs obtained at the time of injury with a medial malleolus and fibula fracture and disruption of the syndesmosis. (B) Radiographs taken 2 months after open reduction and internal fixation. There is lateral displacement of the talus with widening of the medial joint space and lack of reduction of the ankle syndesmosis. (C) Radiographs taken 18 months after index injury shows advanced degenerative changes of the ankle secondary to joint incongruency.

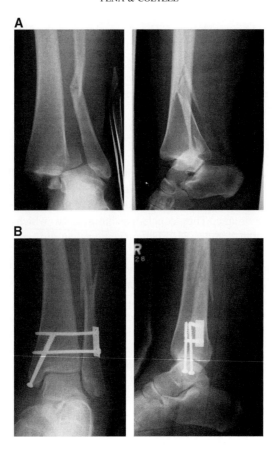

Fig. 2. (*A*) Pronation external rotation injury to the ankle with a syndesmosis disruption. (*B*) After open reduction and internal fixation of the medial malleolus and fixation of the syndesmosis.

load protocol was applied followed by a test to failure. There was no difference in the mechanical behavior of the screws; therefore, mechanically, a bioabsorbable screw is a reasonable alternative.

Hovis and colleagues [24] reported the results of 23 patients after reduction and fixation of the syndesmosis with a 4.5-mm bioabsorbable screw. Postoperatively, the patients were treated with 6 weeks of nonweight bearing that was followed by a program of physical therapy. The investigators reported no malunion, nonunion, or loss of reduction of the syndesmosis or any complications that were related to the biomechanical or biochemical properties of the bioabsorbable screws. Of the 70% of patients who were available for follow-up for a minimum of 24 months, 83% had excellent results and 17% had good results using the Olerud and Molander outcome tool for ankle fractures.

Thornes and colleagues [25] studied a new method of fixation for syndesmosis which included a suture–button construction. Sixteen patients were followed prospectively for 12 months and were compared with a control group that underwent screw fixation. The investigators reported that a faster return to work was associated with the suture–button fixation and no complications occurred with that system. All patients showed a well-maintained reduction on the CT scan findings at 3 months. The randomization process was based on the surgeon's preference and technique.

The TightRope (Arthrex Inc., Naples, Florida) was designed to maintain reduction of the syndesmosis while allowing motion of the fibula with respect to the tibia in a rotational and proximal–distal plane. To place the TightRope, a 3.5-mm hole is drilled across the syndesmosis from lateral to medial at approximately 1 cm to 2 cm above the ankle joint line. The TightRope is passed across the tibia in the same direction. After the medial button on it reaches the medial cortex of the tibia, the button is flipped and is placed flat against the cortex. The button must lay flat against the cortex without any soft tissue interposition to avoid subsequent loosening of the construction. Tension in the suture loads across the medial and lateral button maintains reduction of the syndesmosis. Tension is obtained by suturing tightly over the lateral button (Fig. 3).

Some investigators advocate ankle arthroscopy when reducing an ankle fracture. This assists in the identification of associated injuries and helps to assess the reduction and necessity of addressing the syndesmosis joint surgically (Figs. 4–7).

Treatment of chronic injuries

In the presence of hypertrophic scar tissue, ankle arthroscopy is recommended to assess the joint and to remove scar tissue from the medial gutter and syndesmosis. From the ankle joint it can be reached up to 1 to 1.5 cm proximally into the syndesmosis recess.

Ogilvie-Harris and Reed [26] reported on 17 patients who had chronic syndesmosis injuries that were evaluated and treated arthroscopically. Preoperatively, all of the patients had a positive external rotation stress test. At the time of arthroscopy, the investigators reported clear visualization of the posterior and anterior inferior tibiofibular ligaments and the interosseous ligament. They assessed the instability of the syndesmosis by probing the tibiofibular joint and looking for any gapping in excess of 2 mm. In the presence of instability, debridement of the syndesmosis area with a 3.5-mm soft tissue resector was performed. No fixation was used. The patients participated in a physical therapy program for at least 3 months. All patients required resection of the remaining interosseous ligament; the ligament protruded into the joint 1 mm to 4 mm. Pain was improved in 50% of the patients and stiffness was improved in 25% of the patients. Half of the patients were examined postoperatively; the external rotation stress test did not produce any further pain. Fixation of the syndesmosis may have improved these results.

Harper [27] reported on the reconstruction of failed syndesmosis fixation from 2003. The investigator described a 1-year follow-up, using the American Orthopaedic Foot and Ankle Society outcome score, on six patients who had

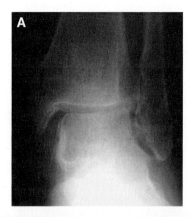

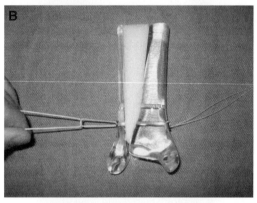

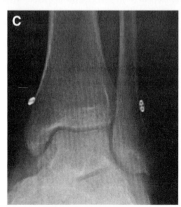

Fig. 3. (*A*) Anteroposterior (AP) view of a widened syndesmosis. (*B*) TightRope system for syndesmosis fixation. (*C, D*) AP and lateral weight-bearing radiographs 6 months after a TightRope fixation of a syndesmosis disruption.

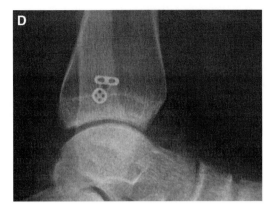

Fig. 3 (*continued*).

recurrent widening of the syndesmosis. Two patients required debridement of the tibiofibular interspace and two patients required debridement of the medial gutter and the tibiofibular interspace. Syndesmosis fixation constructs included 4.5-mm to 7.3-mm cannulated screws that engaged three or four cortices. A well-reduced and maintained reduction occurred in all but one case. On CT scan assessment, function was related to the quality of reduction. The one patient with a poor outcome had failure of the reconstruction. The investigator em-

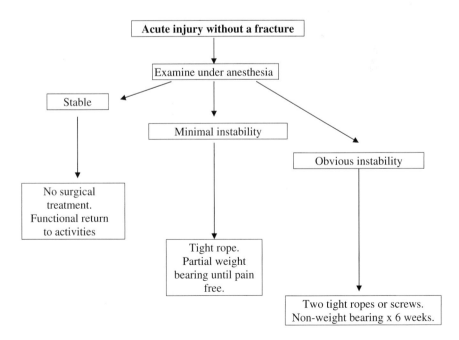

Fig. 4. Algorithm for ankle syndemosis injuries in the absence of a fracture.

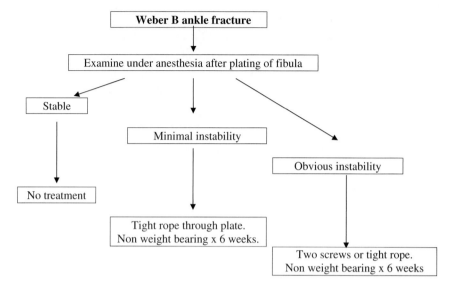

Fig. 5. Algorithm for ankle syndemosis injuries in the presence of a Weber B ankle fracture.

phasized the possibility of accurate diagnosis and reduction of such a chronic injury, and the possibility of restoring the ankle mechanics through a stable and sturdy construction.

Grass and colleagues [28] reported on 16 patients who underwent reconstruction of the syndesmosis ligaments using an autogenous peroneus longus tendon graft. The reconstruction reproduced the three main soft tissue restrainers of the ankle syndesmosis. The peroneus brevis tendon could not be used because of its short length. The patients were allowed partial weight bearing for the first 8 weeks. No rigid fixation was used to maintain reduction of the syndesmosis. The average Karlsson score was 88. Ninety-four percent of the patients were

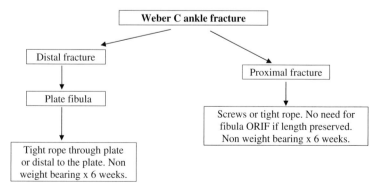

Fig. 6. Algorithm for ankle syndemosis injuries in the presence of a Weber C ankle fracture.

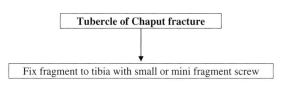

Fig. 7. Algorithm for ankle syndemosis injuries in the presence of a fracture of Chaput's tubercle.

pain-free after an average of 16 months. The radiographic parameters of the ankle syndesmosis improved as there was a more congruent ankle syndesmosis.

Special situations for ankle syndesmosis

Synostosis

The presence of a synostosis in the syndesmosis may cause future disability that is secondary to pain or stiffness of the ankle joint. In a retrospective study, Taylor and colleagues [29] reported the findings on 50 syndesmosis injuries in 44 football players. Fifty percent of those who had radiographs developed heterotopic ossification within the interosseous membrane that prolonged the recovery time.

The reason for a synostosis of the ankle syndesmosis after an injury is not clear. The pathophysiology of heterotopic ossification continues to be unknown. Similarly, it is difficult to propose any treatment to avoid heterotopic ossification or synostosis.

Kottmeier and colleagues [30] reported a case report of a fibula stress fracture in a patient who had synostosis of the ankle syndesmosis. Bostman [31] reported a slightly higher prevalence of synostosis within the ankle syndesmosis after the use of bioabsorbable implants. The biologic environment that is created by alpha-hydroxy polyester may promote heterotopic bone and syndesmosis.

The prevalence of an ankle syndesmosis synostosis after an ankle fracture has been reported between to range between 1.7% and 18.2% [32–35].

Ankle syndesmosis fusion

Surgical technique

An ankle syndesmosis fusion may be performed through an anterolateral approach. Soft tissues are stripped from the medial distal fibula and the most lateral tibia. The most distal margin of the fusion site should be 1 cm proximal to the joint line. The lateral cortex of the tibia and the medial cortex of the fibula are stripped and pushed posteriorly for a total extension of 2 cm to 3 cm (or 3–4 cm from the joint line). Special attention has to be paid to avoid any disruption of the articular surface of the ankle which could create a stress raiser along the most distal portion of the tibia with subsequent collapse of the articular surface. A large amount of bone graft is packed into the site, and two syndesmosis screws are placed across the joint. It is ideal to place a small bone block between the tibia and fibula to prevent narrowing of the ankle mortise when the screws are inserted. A one-third semitubular plate helps to compress the syndesmosis by applying a buttress effect and avoids any widening of the most distal fibula. Postoperatively, the patient is maintained nonweight bearing until radiographic fusion is visualized—approximately the eighth to tenth postoperative week.

Outcome

The outcome of an ankle syndesmosis fusion is not reported in the English literature. Although it is an excellent option as a salvage procedure, it must be emphasized that patient satisfaction is related directly to the preoperative pain and disability. It is the authors' perception that final ankle function after the distal tibiofibular joint motion is obliterated is acceptable for activities of daily living,

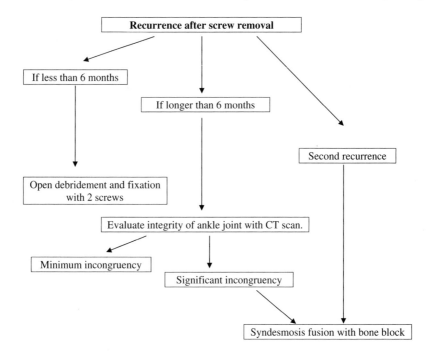

Screw removal: Never before 6 months
                         Four cortices to allow removal of medial broken fragment

Fig. 8. Algorithm for ankle syndemosis injuries for recurrence of syndemosis instability after screw removal.

but it definitely is not sufficient to maintain an active athletic life. Therefore, only the most disabled patient is satisfied with such an intervention (Figs. 3–8).

References

[1] Hopkinson WJ, Pierre PS, Ryan JB, et al. Syndesmosis sprains of the ankle. Foot Ankle 1990; 10(6):325–30.

[2] Fallat L, Grimm MS, Saracco JA. Sprained ankle syndrome: prevalence and analysis of 639 acute injuries. J Foot Ankle Surg 1998;37:280–5.

[3] Boytin MJ, Fischer DA, Nemann L. Syndesmotic ankle sprains. Am J Sports Med 1991;19(3): 294–8.

[4] Karrholm J, Hansson LI, Selvik G. Mobility of the lateral malleolus. Acta Othop Scand 1985; 56:479–83.

[5] Beumer A, Valstar ER, Garling EH, et al. Kinematics of the distal tibiofibular syndesmosis. Radiostereometry in 11 normal ankles. Acta Orthop Scand 2003;74:337–43.

[6] Ogilvie-Harris DJ, Reed SC, Hedman TP. Disruption of the ankle syndesmosis: biomechanical study of the ligamentous restraints. Arthroscopy 1994;10:558–60.

[7] Xenos JS, Hopkinson WJ, Mulligan ME, et al. The tibiofibular syndesmosis. Evaluation of the ligamentous structures, methods of fixation, and radiographic assessment. J Bone Joint Surg Am 1995;77:847–56.

[8] Pereira DS, Koval KJ, Resnick RB, et al. Tibiotalar contact area and pressure distribution: the effect of mortise widening and syndesmosis fixation. Foot Ankle Int 1996;17:269–74.

[9] Alonso A, Khoury L, Adams R. Clinical tests for ankle syndesmosis injury: reliability and prediction of return to function. J Orthop Sports Phys Ther 1998;27:276–84.

[10] Kiter E, Bozkurt M. The crossed-leg test for examination of ankle syndesmosis injuries. Foot Ankle Int 2005;19:187–8.

[11] Teitz CC, Harrington RM. A biomechanical analysis of the squeeze test for sprains of the syndesmotic ligaments of the ankle. Foot Ankle Int 1998;19:489–92.

[12] Beumer A, Valstar ER, Garling EH, et al. External rotation stress imaging in syndesmotic injuries of the ankle. Comparison of lateral radiography and radiostereometry in a cadaveric model. Acta Orthop Scand 2003;74:201–5.

[13] Beumer A, van Hemert WLW, Niesing R, et al. Radiographic measurement of the distal tibio-fibular syndesmosis has limited use. Clin Orthop 2004;423:227–34.

[14] Brown KW, Morrison WB, Schweitzer ME, et al. MRI findings associated with distal tibiofibu-lar syndesmosis injury. AJR Am J Roentgenol 2004;182:131–6.

[15] Ebraheim NA, Lu J, Yang H, et al. Radiographic and CT evaluation of tibiofibular syndes-motic diastasis: a cadaver study. Foot Ankle Int 1997;18:693–8.

[16] Thordarson DB, Motamed S, Hedman T, et al. The effect of fibular malreduction on contact pressures in an ankle fracture malunion model. J Bone Joint Surg 1997;79A(12):1809–15.

[17] Takao M, Ochi M, Naito K, et al. Arthroscopic diagnosis of tibiofibular syndesmosis disruption. Arthroscopy 2001;17:836–43.

[18] Tornetta P, Spoo JE, Reynolds FA, et al. Overtightening of the ankle syndesmosis: is it really possible? J Bone Joint Surg Am 2001;83-A:489–92.

[19] McBryde A, Chiasson B, Wilhelm A, et al. Syndesmotic screw placement: a biomechanical analysis. Foot Ankle Int 1997;18:262–6.

[20] Thompson MC, Gesink DS. Biomechanical comparison of syndesmosis fixation with 3.5- and 4.5-millimeter stainless steel screws. Foot Ankle Int 2000;21:736–41.

[21] Hoiness P, Stromsoe K. Tricortical versus quadricortical syndesmosis fixation in ankle fractures. A prospective, randomized study comparing two methods of syndesmosis fixation. J Orthop Trauma 2004;18:331–7.

[22] Beumer A, Campo MM, Niesing R, et al. Screw fixation of the syndesmosis: a cadaver

model comparing stainless steel and titanium screws and three and four cortical fixation. Injury 2005;36:60–4.

[23] Cox S, Mukherjee DP, Ogden AL, et al. Distal tibiofibular syndesmosis fixation: a cadaveric, simulated fracture stabilization study comparing bioabsorbable and metallic single screw fixation. J Foot Ankle Surg 2005;44:144–51.

[24] Hovis WD, Kaiser BW, Watson JT, et al. Treatment of syndesmotic disruptions of the ankle with bioabsorbable screw fixation. J Bone Joint Surg Am 2002;84A:26–31.

[25] Thornes B, Shannon F, Guiney A-M, et al. Suture-button syndesmosis fixation. Clin Orthop 2005;431:207–12.

[26] Ogilvie-Harris DJ, Reed SC. Disruption of the ankle syndesmosis: diagnosis and treatment by arthroscopic surgery. Arthroscopy 1994;10:561–8.

[27] Harper MC. Delayed reduction and stabilization of the tibiofibular syndesmosis. Foot Ankle Int 2001;22:15–8.

[28] Grass R, Rammelt S, Biewener A, et al. Peroneus longus ligamentoplasty for chronic instability of the distal tibiofibular syndesmosis. Foot Ankle Int 2003;24(5):392–7.

[29] Taylor DC, Englehardt DL, Bassett III FH. Syndesmosis sprains of the ankle. The influence of heterotopic ossification. Am J Sports Med 1992;20:146–50.

[30] Kottmeier SA, Hanks GA, Kalenak A. Fibular stress fracture associated with distal tibiofibular synostosis in an athlete. A case report and literature review. Clin Orthop 1991;281:195–8.

[31] Bostman OM. Distal tibiofibular synostosis after malleolar fractures treated using absorbable implants. Foot Ankle 1993;14:38–43.

[32] Kaye RA. Stabilization of ankle syndesmosis injuries with a syndesmosis screw. Foot Ankle 1989;9(6):290–3.

[33] Wilson FC, Skilbred A. Long-term results in the treatment of displaced bimalleolar fractures. J Bone Joint Surg 1966;48A(6):1065–78.

[34] Cedell CA. Supination-outward rotation injuries to the ankle. Acta Orthop Scand 1967; Suppl 110:103–16.

[35] Phillips WA, Schwartz HS, Keller CS, et al. A prospective randomized study of the management of severe ankle fractures. J Bone Joint Surg 1985;67A(1):67–78.

ELSEVIER
SAUNDERS

Foot Ankle Clin N Am
11 (2006) 51–60

FOOT AND
ANKLE CLINICS

Reconstruction of Failed Ankle Fractures

W. Bryce Henderson, MD, Johnny T.C. Lau, MD, MSc*

*University Health Network, Toronto Western Hospital, Department of Surgery, University of Toronto,
339 Bathurst Street, 1 East Wing – 438, Toronto, Ontario M5T 2S8, Canada*

Ankle fractures are some of the most common injuries that are treated by orthopedic surgeons. Optimal long-term results of ankle fractures require accurate reconstruction, a thorough understanding of the mechanism of injury, and accurate radiographic assessment. Failure to reduce and maintain fractures and dislocations around the ankle properly predisposes to instability and late osteoarthritis. This article focuses on the reconstruction of failed ankle reconstruction that results in malunion or nonunion. The indications for fusion or arthroplasty to treat end-stage degenerative changes are discussed. The treatment of concomitant infection and neuropathic fractures are outlined.

Radiographic analysis

Radiographic assessment of ankle fractures includes measurement of radiographic parameters for accepted reduction. The medial clear space, talocrural angle, tibia–fibula clear space, and lateral talar shift have been correlated independently with poor overall outcome after ankle fracture reduction [1]. Malunion of the medial malleolus is less common than fibular malunion. Unrecognized syndesmotic injury usually can be seen radiographically and clinically. A lack of standardization for radiographic magnification makes absolute measurement of displacement distances unreliable.

Medial clear space—the distance between the medial malleolus and the talus at the level of the syndesmosis—has been related to poor long-term results if greater than 4 mm [2]. In mechanical stress studies, lateral talar shift of more than 1 mm caused articular incongruity. This is due to the loss of congruency of ar-

* Corresponding author.
E-mail address: johnny.lau@utoronto.ca (J.T.C. Lau).

1083-7515/06/$ – see front matter © 2006 Elsevier Inc. All rights reserved.
doi:10.1016/j.fcl.2005.12.006

foot.theclinics.com

ticulating surfaces and a decrease in contact surface area of the joint as the talus shifts laterally [3].

Analysis of the talocrural angle allows one to judge the length of the fibular reduction compared with the medial malleolus. The talocrural angle is the angle between the perpendicular from the distal tibial articular surface and a line from the tips of the medial and lateral malleoli. The talocrural angle is $83° \pm 4°$, but should be compared with the opposite, noninjured ankle [4]. Talar tilt is the angle between a line parallel to the upper surface of the talus and a line parallel to the long axis of the tibia. Talar tilt is less than $5°$ but should be compared with the opposite, noninjured side. The most accurate and reproducible radiographic tool to demonstrate ankle instability is the comparison of medial clear space to the width of the ankle joint space between the superior surface of the talus and the inferior surface of the tibia [5]. A larger medial than superior clear space illustrates instability and is internally controlled for magnification when comparisons are made on the same radiograph.

Analysis of the lateral side of the ankle is more complicated. Assessment of syndesmotic injury, rotation of the fibula, and fibular length should be considered. Fibular rotation is difficult to visualize on plain radiographs. A widened tibia–fibular clear space or subtle fibula fracture malalignment may be the only radiographic evidence of malreduction [6]. A CT scan is used to routinely assess fibular clear space, fracture fragment reduction, and rotation of the distal fragment in cases where adequate reduction has not been achieved. The radiographic tibiofibular clear space should be less than 5 mm on any view, and is the distance between the medial border of the fibula and the incisura border of the distal lateral tibia 1 cm above the ankle [1]. Tibia and fibular overlap between the medial border of the fibula and the lateral border of the tibia on the anteroposterior view is another radiographic measure of the syndesmotic reduction. This value is abnormal if less than 10 mm [1].

Approach to management

Management of a previously injured ankle fracture with respect to malreduction, nonunion, malunion, or osteoarthritis has not been defined clearly. Variables that affect treatment include elapsed time since the injury, severity of injury, success of reduction or fixation, presence of degenerative arthritis, and patient symptoms. Some patients may develop symptoms much later. The optimal time to perform reconstruction for malunions has not been defined clearly. The amount of arthritis complicates the scenario because it may prevent symptom resolution after corrective osteotomy or reconstruction. Patients may continue to improve up to 7 years after reconstruction, even in the presence of mild arthritis [7]. Reconstructive surgery can decrease symptoms of arthritis by decreasing instability and load on the arthritic portion of the joint. Reconstruction may reduce the progression of degenerative change. Patients may require ankle replacement or fusion in the future, despite improved overall alignment and joint congruity. Patients who have chronic infection or severe neuropathy will be better served with an arthrodesis.

Malunion and nonunion of medial malleolus

Fractures of the medial malleolus can vary from simple large fragments to comminuted multiple fragments that are difficult to reduce anatomically. Fractures also can be isolated to the malleolus or can extend into the tibial plafond. Ankle injuries are caused by a rotational force, whereas distal tibial fractures and plafond fractures are caused by an impacting force in the sagittal plane [5]. Assessment of reduction may require a preoperative and postoperative CT scan. Open reduction of bimalleolar fractures is superior to closed reduction. Nonanatomic reduction of the medial malleolar fragment does not affect outcome [7].

Failure to unite after 4 to 6 months results in nonunion [8]. Patients may complain of pain, instability, or have persistent swelling that is related to the pseudarthrosis. Infection, osteochondritis dissecans, posterior tibial tendon syndrome, chondral injury, and tarsal tunnel syndrome may cause medial pain after an ankle fracture. Physical examination, a thorough history, and investigations, including MRI or CT scan, help to determine the correct diagnosis.

Reconstruction of medial malleolar nonunions resulted in a 50% union rate [9]. Difficulty in achieving union can be related to poor fixation, bone loss that is due to comminution, and large amounts of scar from previous operations.

Anatomic reduction under direct visualization is the goal of primary and revision surgery. An incision over the anterior border of the medial malleolus or a curved incision that extends medially allows visualization of the articular surface of the tibial plafond and the medial "shoulder" of the ankle. Smaller fragments can be excised, however no reports of fragment size appropriate for excision have been indentified. Reduction of larger fragments should be anatomic if at all possible. A "Shentons line of the ankle" has been previously described by Weber and Simpson and describes the dense subchondral bone from the medial malleolus, across the tibial plafond extending down across the syndesmosis to the lateral articulation between the fibula and the talar body [13]. This dense bone can be used to guide large fragment reduction radiographically. Internal fixation with screws is usually necessary and a buttress plate is advised if a vertical component is present in the plane of the fracture. The authors routinely fix medial malleolus fractures with two small-fragment cancellous screws. Pilon fractures are plated on the medial side through an open technique and bone graft is added to fill any areas of cancellous defect. Bone graft usually is not necessary for isolated medial malleolus fractures, and is difficult to contain in the area of the nonunion. If the residual fragment is too small for a screw a k-wire can be used in association with a tension-band wire.

When fixation cannot be achieved, fragment removal with advancement of the deltoid to bone with drill holes or suture anchors can be done to improve medial side stability.

Postoperatively, the authors keep all patients nonweight bearing for 6 weeks. Range of motion exercises start at 4 weeks. Patients are changed from a plaster splint to an air cast at suture removal.

Nonunion of the posterior malleolus

Previous reports recommended reduction and fixation of posterior malleolus fragments when the piece is at least 25% or greater of the articular surface and is

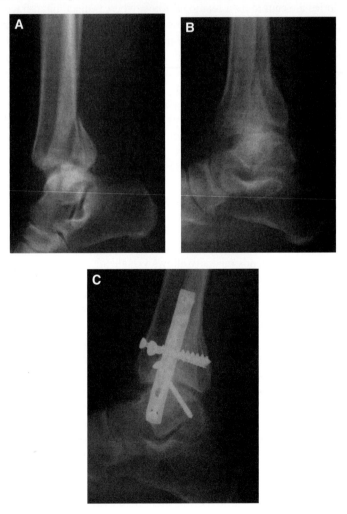

Fig. 1. (*A*) Displaced posterior malleolus fracture. Posterior fragment is greater than 20% of the surface area. (*B*) The patient did not have surgery and the ankle remained subluxed posteriorly because of malunion of the posterior malleolus and fibula fractures. (*C*) Nine months later, the fibula and posterior malleolus were osteotomized and reduced anatomically.

displaced with a 3-mm gap or 2-mm step deformity [9]. These criteria are based on plain films and can be seen more clearly on CT scan.

Posterior malleolus injuries rarely occur in isolation. Usually, they are associated with medial and lateral injuries. The intact posterior tibia–fibular ligament indirectly reduces the posterior malleolus with reduction of the fibula. The presence of a posterior malleolar fragment indicates a more severe injury and an increased incidence of ankle arthritis [10].

Conflicting data on the outcome of posterior malleolar reduction exists. Harper and Hardin [11] showed no clinical benefit from reducing the posterior malleolus after anatomic reduction of the medial and lateral malleolus. Mont and colleagues [1] found that patients who had a larger posterior malleolar fracture had a worse result.

Posterior malleolar fractures that are greater than 20% of the articular surface should be reduced anatomically (Fig 1A). This usually occurs with anatomic reduction of the fibula fracture. If not, open reduction and fixation with a screw is required. The reduction can be visualized through the fractured fibula and a single screw is placed anterior to posterior. Alternatively, the posterior malleolus is reached posterior to the transfixed fibula and held with posterior to anterior screws. A cannulated screw can be used. When the posterior malleolar fragment is very large the fracture can be approached through the medial malleolar fracture (Fig 1B, C). A formal posteromedial or posterolateral approach is performed in revision cases where the medial or lateral malleoli are intact. The fragment is mobilized and reduced under direct vision and fixed with one or two cancellous screws. Bone graft and buttress plating are used only if there is fragment comminution or if the surgeon is not satisfied with interfragmentary screw fixation.

Fibular malunion

Malunion of the fibula is the most common and most difficult nonunion to reconstruct. Malunion may be secondary to nonunion or errors in properly reconstructing rotation and length of the fractured fibula. Osteopenia in the distal fibular fragment complicates the reconstruction. Care must be taken to reduce the fibula into the syndesmosis and to reduce the talus against the medial malleolus. Occasionally, it is necessary to open the ankle medially to remove scar, deltoid ligament, or cartilage flaps that is preventing reduction.

To regain length of the fibula, the talocrural angle should be restored to the same as in the normal ankle. A transverse or oblique osteotomy allows distal transport of the fibula. An oblique osteotomy through the original fracture allows better correction but it is more difficult to do. The transverse osteotomy is performed proximal to the syndesmosis. A transverse osteotomy allows for correction of length and rotation. A lamina spreader can be used to distract the proximal and distal fragments, and k-wires are inserted into the tibia until a structural bone graft is placed (Fig. 2). It is transfixed with a one-third semitubular plate. Intraoperative radiographs are used to judge length and reduction. Direct observation

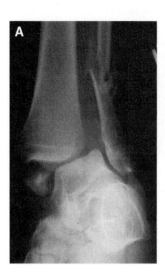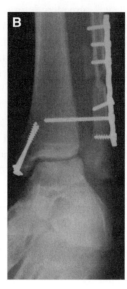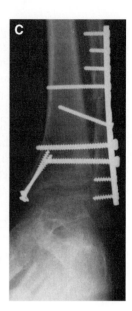

Fig. 2. (*A*) Bimalleolar ankle fracture with fibula comminution. (*B*) Fibula fracture was fixed short and externally rotated. (*C*) Six weeks later, the fibula malunion was corrected with a transverse osteotomy proximal to syndesmosis, structural iliac crest autograft, derotation, and fixation of osteotomy and syndesmosis.

of the lateral articular facet of the fibula can assist in assessment of reduction. Reduction of the fibula also should be assessed by direct visualization of the syndesmosis.

Internal rotation of the distal fibular fragment is necessary to reduce the rotational deformity of the fracture correctly (Fig. 3). A lateral plate in 10° of internal rotation corrects external rotation deformity of the distal fragment [12].

Choices of bone graft vary between structural allograft, iliac crest structural autograft, and cancellous autograft [13]. Soft tissue closure over the plate and bone graft may be difficult when more than 1 cm of length is obtained because soft tissues can be contracted.

Postoperatively, patients are placed in a plaster backslab with the foot in neutral and are kept nonweight bearing for 6 weeks. At 2 weeks the sutures are removed and they are changed to an air cast. At 4 weeks they are allowed to move their ankle actively.

Syndesmotic widening

The syndesmotic articulation between the tibia and the fibula is maintained by the anterior tibiofibular ligament, the posterior tibiofibular ligament, and the interosseous ligament. The injury to the syndesmosis in Weber B– and C-type

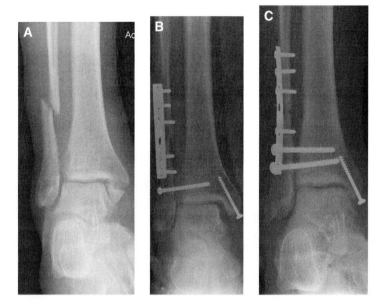

Fig. 3. (*A*) Bimalleolar ankle fracture with fibula fracture above syndesmosis. (*B*) Bimalleolar ankle fracture was treated with open reduction and internal fixation. The fibula fracture is malreduced with a mismatch of the width of cortices at the level of the fibula fracture, which indicates an external rotation malunion. The external rotation produces a lateral talar shift. (*C*) The fibula fracture was revised 6 weeks later by rotating the distal fragment internally and stabilizing the syndesmosis.

injuries requires reduction and stabilization [6]. The syndesmosis reduction should be anatomic for good outcome [2].

The syndesmosis should be examined directly during open reduction of ankle fractures. Direct visualization of the syndesmosis can be performed with adequate exposure and dorsiflexion and eversion of the ankle. Lateral displacement of the distal fibula indicates instability. Alternatively, C-arm stress views are performed. The proximal tibia is held by an assistant and the ankle is rotated externally. Any lateral displacement of the talus or distal fibular confirms an unstable syndesmosis. Recommended fixation involves noncannulated fully threaded cortical screws through four cortices; this allows for easier late removal in case of screw breakage. The patient may begin ankle range of motion exercises starting at 6 weeks but should remain non weight bearing for 12 weeks.

For patients who have a missed syndesmotic injury, talar displacement or talar tilt requires revision surgery. A CT scan or MRI assists in identifying any degenerative changes or scar in the syndesmosis that is to be removed at the time of syndesmotic fixation. The screw is placed through the lateral plate. If the syndesmosis requires debridement the dissection is taken anteriorly over the fibula to access the syndesmotic articulation. The authors usually do not graft the syndesmosis, replace the syndesmotic ligament, or attempt a tibiofibular synostosis.

Degenerative changes

Thirty-three percent of patients who have Weber B– and C-type fractures have persistent symptoms [10] that may be secondary to the cartilage damage that occurs in 12% of routine ankle fractures [14]. Investigation may include MRI or CT; however, ankle arthroscopy is the best method for joint assessment. Debridement and hardware removal can be performed at the same time as ankle

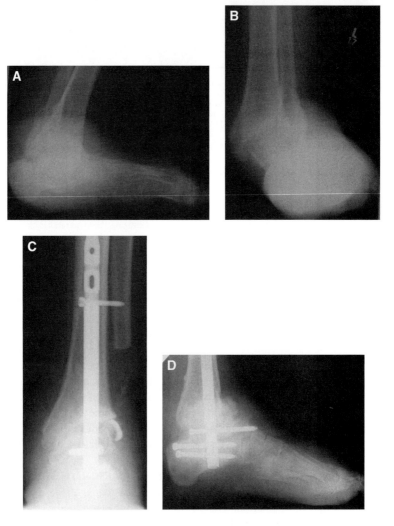

Fig. 4. Lateral (*A*) and anteroposterior (*B*) radiographs of a collapsed neuropathic ankle with fibula fracture. Poor bone stock, deformity, and soft tissue swelling are evident. Anteroposterior (*C*) and lateral (*D*) radiographs of the neuropathic ankle fracture that was treated by tibiotalar fusion with a retrograde intramedullary nail.

arthroscopy. Patients who have ankle fractures and degenerative changes should be treated initially with anti-inflammatory medications and a noncustom ankle brace. With more severe changes, a custom ankle foot orthosis with a rocker bottom sole is recommended. Surgical options are discussed, including ankle replacement, ankle fusion, and cheilectomy, after patients have maximized their nonoperative treatment. Ankle fusion remains the standard treatment for post-traumatic ankle arthritis in young patients. Ankle arthroplasty shows moderate success, but has a higher rate of reoperation and failure than does hip or knee arthroplasty [11]. Ankle replacement is contraindicated in the presence of active or recent infection, neuropathic joint, osteonecrosis of the talus, severe mal-alignment, vascular impairment, a compromised soft tissue envelope, severe joint laxity, and neurologic dysfunction of the lower extremity [8].

Infection and neuropathy

Infection and neuropathy complicate the fixation and healing of fractures. Chronic osteomyelitis or infection may require intravenous antibiotics and re-moval of implants with external or fine-wire fixation. All acute (<3 months since index procedure) infections are treated with intravenous antibiotics followed by oral antibiotics and hardware is retained. Patients who have evidence of abscess or suppuration are taken to the operating room for irrigation and debridement, with retention of implants. Proceeding to ankle fusion may be prudent if future surgeries place the skin and soft tissues at further risk. Fractures that are com-plicated by severe neuropathy may require early ankle fusion, especially if bone quality precludes bony fixation and difficulty maintaining reduction (Fig. 4A, B). Primary ankle fusion for severe ankle or distal tibia fractures has results that are inferior to early fixation and late fusion [14–18]. Severely neuropathic patients who have ankle or fracture instability may ulcerate, develop osteomyelitis, or require amputation. In these cases a stable plantigrade foot and ankle may only be achieved with an ankle fusion (Fig. 4C, D). In the presence of active infection, an external fixation type of fusion is warranted.

Summary

Operative fixation of ankle fractures is a routine procedure for many ortho-pedic surgeons. Malunion of medial, lateral, or posterior malleoli may present in the early or late postoperative period. Anatomic reduction of all components of the fractured ankle is the goal of reconstructive surgery. Failure to reduce and maintain the syndesmosis properly results in poor outcome. Degenerative changes can result from damage to the articular surface at the time of injury, or from an improperly reduced syndesmosis or malleolus increasing joint wear which results in an arthritic ankle joint. Ultimately, ankle fusion or replacement may be required in an arthritic ankle when nonoperative measures have failed.

Attention to the factors that were outlined in this paper will help to decrease the number of ankle reconstructions that are required after ankle fracture treatment.

References

[1] Mont M, Sedlin E, Weiner L, et al. Postoperative radiographs as predictors of clinical outcome in unstable ankle fractures. J Orthop Trauma 1992;6(3):352–7.

[2] McDaniel WJ, Wilson FC. Trimalleolar fractures of the ankle. An end result study. Clin Orthop 1977;122:37–45.

[3] Michelson JD. Ankle fractures resulting from rotational injuries. J Am Acad Orthop Surg 2003; 11(6):403–13.

[4] Ramsey PL, Hamilton W. Changes in tibiotalar area of contact caused by lateral talar shift. J Bone Joint Surg 1976;58A(3):356–7.

[5] Marti RK, Raaymakers EL, Nolte PA. Malunited ankle fractures. The late results of recon-struction. J Bone Joint Surg 1990;72B(4):709–13.

[6] Spirit AA, Assal M, Hansen ST. Complications after total ankle arthoplasty. J Bone J Surg 2004;86(6):1172–8.

[7] Kelikian AS, Kelikian H. Aspects of tibial malleolar fractures. In: Kelikian AS, editor. Disorders of the ankle. Philadelphia: WB Saunders; 1985. p. 287–338.

[8] Rhys HT, Daniels TR. Ankle arthritis. J Bone Joint Surg 2003;85:923–36.

[9] Rockwood CA, Green DP, Bucholz RW, et al. Fractures in adults. Vol. 2. Philadelphia: Lippincott-Raven; 1996.

[10] Lindsjo U. Operative treatment of ankle fracture-dislocations. A follow up study of 306/321 consecutive cases. Clin Orthop 1985;199:28–38.

[11] Harper MC, Hardin G. Posterior malleolar fractures of the ankle associated with external rotation-abduction injuries. J Bone Joint Surg 1988;70A(9):1348–56.

[12] Sneppen O. Treatment of pseudarthrosis involving the malleolus. A postoperative follow-up of 34 cases. Acta Orthop Scand 1971;42(2):201–16.

[13] Uribe J, Neufeld SK, Myerson MS. Fresh-frozen structural allografts in the foot and ankle. J Bone Joint Surg 2005;87:113–20.

[14] Sarkisian JS, Cody GW. Closed treatment of ankle fractures: a new criterion for evaluation-a review of 250 cases. J Trauma 1976;16(4):323–6.

[15] Stiehl JB. Late reconstruction of ankle fractures and dislocations. In: Gould JS, editor. Operative foot surgery. Philadelphia: WB Saunders; 1994. p. 356–76.

[16] Trafton PG, Bray TJ, Simpson LA. Fractures and soft tissue injuries of the ankle. In: Browner BD, Jupiter JB, Levine AM, et al, editors. Skeletal trauma. Philadelphia: WB Saunders; 1992. p. 1871–957.

[17] Ward AJ, Ackroyd CE, Baker AS. Late lengthening of the fibula for malaligned ankle fractures. J Bone Joint Surg 1990;72B(4):714–7.

[18] Weber BG, Simpson LA. Corrective lengthening osteotomy of the fibula. Clin Orthop 1985;199: 61–7.

ELSEVIER
SAUNDERS

Foot Ankle Clin N Am
11 (2006) 61–84

FOOT AND
ANKLE CLINICS

Reconstruction After Talar Fractures

Stefan Rammelt, MD*, Jörg Winkler, MD,
René Grass, MD, PhD, Hans Zwipp, MD, PhD

*Trauma and Reconstructive Surgery, University Hospital "Carl Gustav Carus,"
Fetscherstr 74, 01307 Dresden, Germany*

The talus, with its contribution to three important joints, plays a pivotal role in overall foot function. Consequently, posttraumatic malalignment, malunions, or nonunions of the talus almost invariably lead to painful functional impairment [1–4]. Malalignment of the talus that is due to inadequate fracture reduction leads to poor results [5–8]. Typical features of malunited talar fractures include varus malalignment of the talar neck that causes shortening and deformity of the medial column. The foot adopts a hindfoot varus, forefoot varus, and adducted position. Frequently, nonunion after talar neck or body fractures causes pain and gradual malposition with joint incongruity. At the joint surface, residual step deformity leads to posttraumatic arthritis. Displaced bone fragments can cause impingement of the posterior tibial tendons, tarsal tunnel, or the sinus tarsi [2,5, 7,9,10]. Malunion rates of the talar neck of up to 47% have been reported, especially after closed reduction of displaced (Hawkins type II) fractures [5,6,10,11]. The most commonly described deformity is a varus malunion of the talar neck [4,5,9]. Fracture malunions and nonunions of the lateral and posterior processes of the talus lead to painful arthritis and warrant surgical revision [8,12].

In numerous cases, after fracture–dislocations of the talus the course is complicated by avascular necrosis (AVN) of the talar body. Although the problem of talar collapse after AVN is well recognized, and numerous treatment strategies are proposed [13], little has been published on the correction of posttraumatic deformities after talar fractures [1,3].

Salvage procedures after talar malunion with symptomatic posttraumatic arthritis include arthrodesis of the ankle, subtalar, or talonavicular joints; triple arthrodesis; total ankle replacement; and tibiocalcaneal arthrodesis with or with-

---

* Corresponding author.
E-mail address: strammelt@hotmail.com (S. Rammelt).

out astragalectomy [2,5,14–21]. In cases of nonunions and malunited talar fractures, delayed anatomic reconstruction seems to be worthwhile if the joint cartilage is viable, and no talar collapse or infection has occurred [1,4,22,23]. This article gives an overview on reconstructive options after talar malunions or nonunions with residual joint displacement after primary treatment.

Pathomechanics of talar malunion

Fractures of the talar neck frequently are associated with medial comminution, probably because of the impaction forces that are exerted by the sustentaculum tali acting as a lever [24]. Varus malalignment results from inadequate reduction because of limited medial exposure or fixation with lag screws. Experimental varus deformity of the talar neck has led to a significant decrease of subtalar motion that results in an inability to evert the foot, internal rotation of the hindfoot, and adduction of the forefoot [9]. In these experiments, there was a direct correlation between the degree of varus malalignment and the change in subtalar motion and foot position. Furthermore, varus malalignment of the hindfoot decreases the mobility of the midtarsal joints and prevents the normal reciprocal relationship between the hindfoot and forefoot [9]. The talonavicular joint rarely is affected directly by talar fracture–dislocations (with the exception of Hawkins type IV fractures) but is injured in talar head fractures, which often are part of midtarsal fracture–dislocations.

Frequently, incomplete reduction of talar fractures also leads to dorsal displacement of the talar body, and results in limited dorsiflexion at the ankle joint [3,5]. Even if the fracture does not extend into the tibiotalar joint, tilting (declination) of the talus secondary to subtalar dislocation leads to incongruity in the ankle joint with loss of dorsiflexion.

Biomechanical investigations on cadaver specimens with pressure-sensitive film showed that simulated malalignment of only 2 mm at the talar neck resulted in significant load redistribution between the posterior, medial, and anterior facets of the subtalar joint [25]. Therefore, even minor residual step-offs may lead to progressive development of posttraumatic arthritis. The prevalence of nonunion after fractures of the talar neck is reported to be between 0% and 10% [1,6,7].

Fractures of the talar processes are seen frequently in the wake of subtalar dislocations or subluxations and are overlooked in a considerable percentage of cases [26–28]. Nonoperative treatment of fractures of the lateral process regularly leads to painful malunions and nonunions, and may lead to subtalar arthritis, which may indicate underlying cartilage injury [8,27]. The posterior process of the talus contributes to the ankle and subtalar joint. If a separate fragment is visible, one has to differentiate between an asymptomatic os trigonum, symptomatic loosening of an os trigonum, malunion, and nonunion after fracture of the posterior process. Malunited fractures of the posterior process of the talus may lead to painful arthritis at the ankle and—more frequently—the subtalar joint [8,26,28].

Patient selection and preoperative planning

Indications for surgical intervention are intractable pain, inability to bear weight, and severe functional impairment—predominantly restricted range of motion in the ankle, subtalar, and midtarsal joints. All of these features almost invariably occur even after minor incongruities of the joint surfaces. Patients also will bear weight on the lateral border of the foot after talar neck nonunions. Long-standing deformities progress to painful posttraumatic arthritis. Patients should be evaluated with respect to activity level, pain, and functional deficit. Clinical examination should focus on the position of the hindfoot and forefoot on weight bearing. The range of motion and discomfort of hindfoot joints are recorded. Nerves and pulses are examined for deficit. Weight-bearing anterior–posterior, dorsal–plantar (20°), and lateral views of both ankles and feet are obtained. A hindfoot alignment view of both feet is obtained [29]. Radiographic evidence of posttraumatic arthritis and AVN, displacement of bones and joints, and quality of bone stock are assessed. Routine leukocyte counts and serum levels of C-reactive protein should be obtained for all patients who are slated for surgery to rule out infection.

CT scans should be obtained in all cases to assess joint incongruities and to allow for precise preoperative planning. If these investigations are suspicious for AVN, MRI should be used to determine its presence and extent. AVN is considered to be "partial" if less than one third of the talar body is involved and "complete" if more than one third of the talar body is affected and leads to talar collapse [1]. A classification for posttraumatic talar deformities (Box 1) was proposed [2]. MRI also can be used to assess the degree of cartilage damage that is present.

In type I to III deformities (malunion or nonunion with minimal AVN), delayed anatomic reconstruction of the talus with preservation of the joints can be attempted in compliant, active patients who have sufficient bone stock. Patients who have type I to III deformities and severe, symptomatic posttraumatic arthritis

---

Box 1. Classification of posttraumatic talar deformities

Type I: malunion or joint displacement
Type II: nonunion with displacement
Type III: types I/II with partial AVN
Type IV: types I/II with complete AVN
Type V: types I/II with septic AVN

From Zwipp H, Rammelt S. [Posttraumatic deformity correction at the foot]. Zentralbl Chir 2003;128(3):219 [in German].

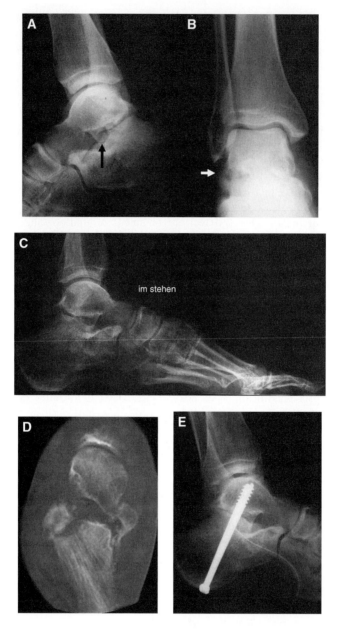

Fig. 1. Malunited fracture of the lateral process of the talus. (*A, B*) A subtalar dislocation with fracture of the lateral process and the sustentaculum tali (*arrows*) was treated nonoperatively. (*C*) The patient presented with painful posttraumatic arthritis of the subtalar joint only 5 months after the injury. (*D*) CT scanning revealed posttraumatic subtalar arthritis at the site of the malunited lateral process fracture and nonunion of the sustentaculum tali. (*E*) In situ fusion of the subtalar joint was performed by way of a lateral oblique (Ollier's) approach. (*F, G*) Significant pain reduction and solid union is noted at 6 months follow-up.

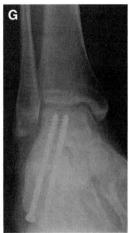

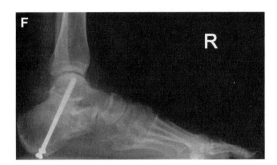

Fig. 1 (*continued*).

can be treated with axial realignment and fusion, while preserving the ankle or subtalar joints if possible. Sometimes, the decision to reconstruct or fuse a joint only can be made intraoperatively while assessing the cartilage status. In patients who have systemic diseases (eg, poorly controlled diabetes mellitus, stage IIb peripheral vascular disease, systemic immune deficiency, severe osteoporosis), secondary anatomic reconstruction may be contraindicated because the risks may outweigh the benefits [1].

Most patients who have complete AVN and collapse of the talar body (type IV malunions) are subjected to tibiotalocalcaneal fusion with autologous bone grafting after excision of necrotic bone. In the presence of osteomyelitis (type V malunions), repeated debridements of infected and necrotic bone almost invariably lead to subtotal talectomy, although in some cases the talar head, and thus, the talonavicular joint may be preserved [19].

In patients who have limited ankle dorsiflexion secondary to dorsal displacement, dorsal beak resection may lead to improved function [5]. Malunions and nonunions after fractures of the lateral or posterior process that lead to joint pain can be salvaged at an early stage by complete excision of the malunited fragments [27,30]. Subtalar joint arthrodesis may be necessary after malunited lateral process fractures and subtalar arthritis. Malunions and nonunions of the posterior process may affect the ankle and subtalar joint. If fusion becomes necessary, the ankle joint should be spared; however, in rare instances a tibiotalocalcaneal fusion may be unavoidable [28]. Because talar process fractures frequently occur after subtalar dislocations, care should be taken to address persistent subluxation in the subtalar joint and to look for associated injuries (eg, fractures of the sustentaculum tali) (Fig. 1).

Secondary anatomic reconstruction

Anatomic reconstruction of talar malunions and nonunions seems to be bene-ficial in young, active patients. They must be compliant enough to restrict weight bearing and be willing to perform an extended protocol of physical therapy to prevent disuse osteopenia.

Surgery is performed with a tourniquet placed at the ipsilateral thigh, and the iliac crest is draped free to allow autologous bone grafting when necessary. Patient position and surgical approach depend on the type and location of the deformity [1]. For malunited fractures of the talar neck an anteromedial approach is used, which allows exposure of the ankle and talonavicular joints. In most instances, the subtalar joint will have to be visualized and an additional anterolateral or oblique lateral (Ollier's) approach is used. The latter also is useful in cases of malunion of the lateral process of the talus. A medial malleolar osteotomy usually is required for correction of malunions of the talar body. In cases of malunited posterior talar body fractures, a posteromedial or posterolateral approach is used.

Careful soft tissue dissection is mandatory. Extensive soft tissue dissection at the tip of the medial malleolus and the inferior aspect of the talar neck has to be avoided to preserve blood supply [31]. To obtain optimal access to the joints, a femoral distractor—placed between the tibia and the calcaneus (Fig. 2)—is extremely helpful, especially in long-standing deformities.

The original fracture line through the talar neck or body is exposed. If the injury is less than 6 weeks old, the fragments are mobilized carefully with a sharp elevator or small osteotome and the fibrous tissue and fracture callus are removed. In most instances, correctional osteotomies need to be made along the former fracture planes. Because the fracture almost invariably extends into the ankle or subtalar joints, care has to be taken to avoid additional cartilage injury. Nonunions require a complete resection of the fibrous pseudarthrosis and scle-rotic bone to viable cancellous bone. The resulting defect requires autologous bone grafting from the ipsilateral iliac crest or tibia.

The quality of the cartilage at the ankle and subtalar joints is assessed by thorough inspection or arthroscopy and probing of all accessible parts (see Fig. 2). If extensive full-thickness cartilage defects of the weight-bearing areas are observed, fusion of the affected joint has to be considered after correction of the deformity. The talonavicular joint mostly is affected indirectly by the deformity and can be preserved in most cases unless an additional injury to the midtarsal joint has taken place [2]. Smaller cartilaginous lesions may be treated with curettage and drilling or microfracturing. Loose, nonviable fragments are excised. The viability of the talar body also is checked with the tourniquet released. Avascular areas of the talar body are subjected to subchondral drilling to enhance bone regeneration; however, if no sclerosis is present, the benefit of this procedure is uncertain [13]. Fibrous intra- and extra-articular adhesions are released and tenolysis is performed, if necessary.

The mobilized fragments are reduced anatomically under direct vision to the ankle and subtalar joint. In cases of nonunion, cancellous bone grafting is

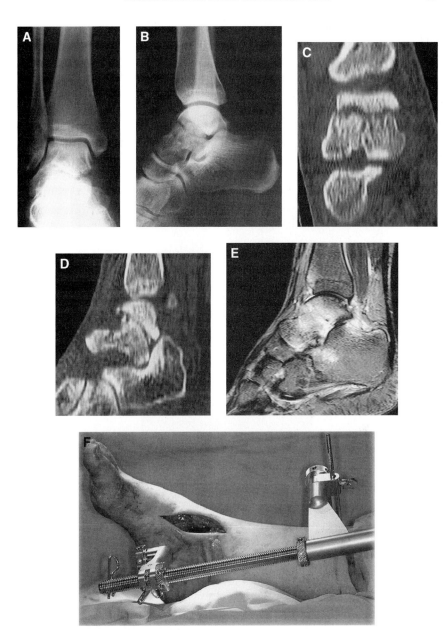

Fig. 2. Reconstruction of a talar malunion without signs of AVN (type I). A 31-year-old woman presented with painful malfunction of the foot 7 weeks after a fall from a horse. The fracture had been treated in a below-knee cast. Radiographs (*A, B*) and CT (*C, D*) revealed a fracture of the talar neck and body with marked dislocation at the subtalar joint. (*E*) A preoperative MRI ruled out AVN. (*F–H*) The subtalar joint was reconstructed using a bilateral approach and a femoral distractor. (*I–L*) The talar body was fixed with 2.7- and 3.5-mm screws. (*M–O*) 18 months after reconstruction no sign of arthritis or AVN is visible. (*P–S*) Range of motion is near normal in the ankle and subtalar joints.

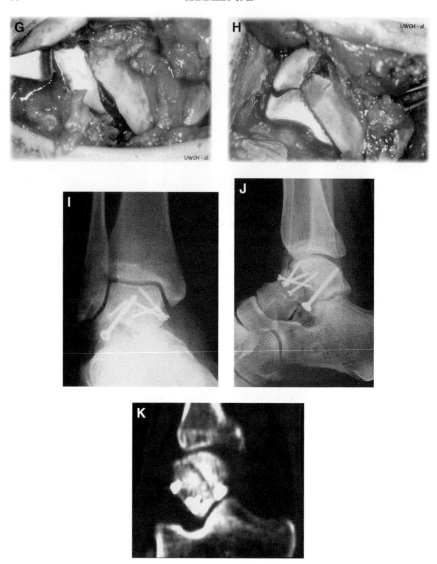

Fig. 2 (*continued*).

necessary after resection of all sclerotic bone to avoid shortening of the talus. If an open wedge osteotomy of the talar neck is performed for varus malunion, a wedge-shaped tricortical corticocancellous graft is used for axial correction [4,23]. After anatomic reconstruction, fragment fixation usually is achieved with 3.5-mm small-fragment titanium screws [1].

Postoperatively, a split nonweight-bearing, below-the-knee cast is applied until swelling subsides. The leg is kept elevated. The cast can be removed temporarily for isometric exercises that are begun at the first postoperative day.

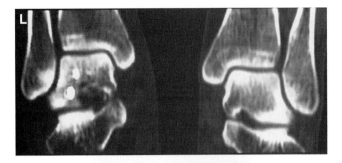

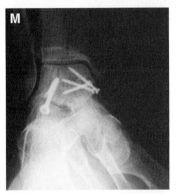

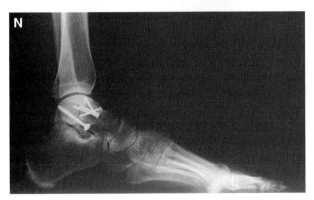

Fig. 2 (*continued*).

Patients are mobilized with crutches under partial weight bearing of 15 to 20 kilograms. Full range-of-motion (ROM) exercises of the ankle, subtalar, and midtarsal joints are initiated on the second postoperative day. After recession of the postoperative edema, patients are protected in an ankle-spanning boot (eg, Variostabil, Adidas Inc., Herzogenaurach, Germany) that can be removed for foot hygiene and ROM exercises. Alternatively, compliant patients may be mobilized with partial weight bearing in their own shoes. Full weight bearing is allowed after radiographic evidence of bone union at an average of 12 weeks

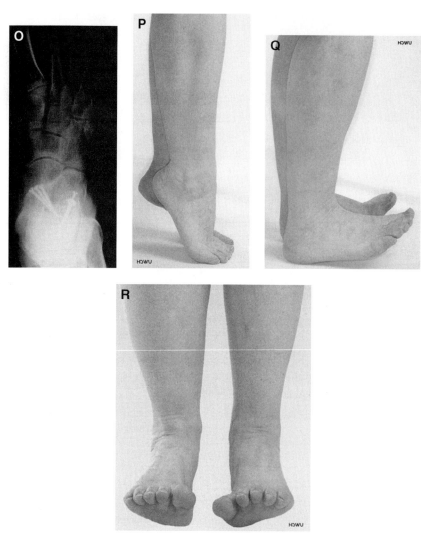

Fig. 2 (*continued*).

postoperatively. The presence of preexisting partial AVN should not prolong the period of partial weight bearing.

Until recently, anatomic reconstruction of the talus after posttraumatic malunion had been reported occasionally [22,32]. Monroe and Manoli [23] successfully corrected one case of malunion of the talar neck by osteotomy and corticocancellous bone grafting. AVN of the talar body did not occur. In his textbook, Hansen [4] described the technique of opening wedge osteotomy for posttraumatic varus malalignment of the talar neck and congenital deformities (eg, clubfoot, cavovarus foot), without reporting any numbers or results. A few investigators reported successful treatment of talar nonunions with bone grafting,

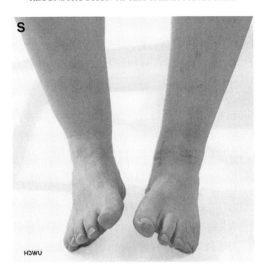

Fig. 2 (*continued*).

but without malalignment and the subsequent necessity of deformity correction [2,4,14,33].

The authors recently reported on 10 patients who were treated over an 8 year-period with secondary anatomic reconstruction for painful incongruities, malunions, or nonunions at a mean of 10 months after sustaining displaced fractures of the talar body or neck [1]. Five patients were classified as having type I malunions, 2 patients were classified as having as type II malunions, and 3 patients were classified as having type III malunions. Correction was performed with osteotomy through the malunited fracture or removal of the pseudarthrosis. Internal fixation was achieved with screws and additional bone grafting, if necessary. No wound healing problems or infections were seen. Solid union was obtained without redislocation in all cases, with no signs of development or progression of AVN. At a mean of 47 months after reconstruction, all patients were satisfied with the result except for 1 patient who required ankle fusion 7.5 years after reconstruction. The mean American Orthopaedic Foot and Ankle Society (AOFAS) ankle hindfoot score increased from 37.7 to 86.2 ($P < .001$). There was no difference in the functional outcome between cases with and without preexisting partial AVN. Three patients who were treated primarily by open reduction and internal fixation, but with residual displacement, had lower AOFAS scores than did the 7 patients who were treated primarily by closed methods or neglected completely (73.7 versus 91.6). Possibly, repeated surgery represented an additional trauma to the soft tissues that resulted in inferior function at follow-up. As a consequence, talar fractures, which are rare injuries, should be treated by surgeons who have appropriate expertise.

Excluding the patient who had late ankle arthrodesis, the ROM was reduced by a mean of 8.5° (range, 0 to 15°) at the ankle and 7.0° (range, 0 to 25°) at the subtalar and midtarsal joints as compared with the unaffected side. On follow-up radiographs, mild, asymptomatic progression of arthritis was noted in the ankle in three cases, and in the subtalar and talonavicular joints in two cases each [1].

Corrective arthrodesis

In cases of severe posttraumatic osteoarthritis secondary to fracture malunion or considerable bone loss after nonunion or AVN, axial realignment and fusion of the affected joint remains a viable salvage option. At the authors' institution, 26 patients were treated with arthrodesis procedures for talar malunions and nonunions during the same period that 10 patients were subjected to secondary reconstruction [1]. In every instance, fusion should be limited to the ankle or subtalar joint. If both have to be fused, every effort should be made to keep the talar head and preserve the talonavicular joint. Arthrodesis must be accompanied by realignment of the anatomic axes of the foot. The surgical approach may be influenced by existing incisions or the state of the soft tissues around the talus. Otherwise, the preferred standard approaches are used for arthrodesis.

Ankle arthrodesis

Numerous options exist for ankle arthrodesis secondary to severe posttraumatic arthritis. In the absence of infection or extended bone loss, internal fixation with screws or plates provides greater stability and higher union rates than does external fixation [34,35]. External fixation devices—temporary or permanent— may be preferable in the presence of infection (type V malunions) [36]. The authors' preference is to perform ankle arthrodesis by way of an anteromedial approach with four screws [35,37].

Several clinical studies showed the best results with ankle fusion in neutral in the coronal plane and neutral to slight valgus (0 to 5°) in the sagittal plane [37–40]. Meticulous care should be taken to correct any deformity that is caused by talar malunion. Coronal plane alignment is achieved by straight resection of the remaining articular cartilage and subchondral sclerotic bone with chisels or an oscillating saw. Significant malalignment is corrected by closed wedge or open wedge osteotomy through the ankle joint plane and a tricortical bone graft, if necessary. The bones are fixed temporarily with Kirschner wires and the exact position of the talus is determined on intraoperative anteroposterior and lateral radiographs of the ankle. Tibiotalar alignment in the sagittal plane is controlled in the lateral radiograph. The angle that is formed by the tibial axis and the inferior aspect of the talus should be no more than 110° to avoid fusion in equinus [39]. Comparison with the unaffected side is useful. Also, the talar dome should be centered exactly beneath the axis of the tibia [37]. A sound arthrodesis usually is achieved with four 6.5-mm cancellous lag screws, or alternatively, cannulated lag screws.

A wealth of clinical studies has reported results after ankle arthrodesis for posttraumatic and idiopathic arthritis. Most were done secondary to malunited malleolar or pilon fractures with no special reference given to talar malunions. Several long-term follow-up studies showed a considerable incidence of subtalar and talonavicular arthritis of between 10% and 100%; the subtalar joint was more affected in most of the studies [38–44]. It seems that some of the observed arthritis of adjacent joints might be related to altered pressure distribution and contact area in these joints after fusion in slight coronal or sagittal malalignment [41,42]; however, not all cases of arthritis that are seen on radiographs become symptomatic. Overall, successful fusion rates and substantial pain relief (80%–100%) have been reported in numerous studies on tibiotalar fusion for ankle arthritis of various causes [37,38,40,43,45,46]. Few reports exist on ankle fusion after talar fractures; all reported substantial pain reduction and functional improvement [14,22,47]. AVN is associated with the risk of nonunion.

Over the last 10 years, total ankle arthroplasty has evolved as an alternative to ankle arthrodesis in cases of severe ankle arthritis [17]. Total ankle replacement is a viable option if the bone stock of the tibia and talus is preserved and no gross deformity is present. The prosthesis may be prone to loosening with partial AVN of the talar dome or a defect within the talar body after removal of a pseudarthrosis; some investigators reported that the talar component is more prone to failure than is the tibial component [48–50]. Although short- and medium-term results of total ankle replacement are encouraging, with the exception of the Scandinavian total ankle replacement design no long-term follow-up exists [51]. There is no reliable arthroplasty option for the subtalar and talonavicular joints. Total ankle replacement is particularly useful if the triple joint complex has to be fused to avoid the complications of a totally stiff ankle/hindfoot complex.

Subtalar arthrodesis

In cases of symptomatic posttraumatic arthritis of the subtalar joint after talar malunion, an in situ arthrodesis with screws over a small posterolateral, anterolateral, or oblique lateral approach usually is effective. In some cases of malunions that affect the ankle and the subtalar joint, the subtalar joint needs to be fused because of loss of cartilage, whereas the ankle joint can be salvaged by realignment of the talar body (Fig. 3). Mahan and Lamy [32] treated one such case of talar neck nonunion with considerable displacement 9 months after the injury with open reduction and internal fixation of the fracture. The ankylosed subtalar joint was fused with autogenous bone grafting, whereas the formerly incongruent ankle joint was preserved. Correctional arthrodesis of the subtalar joint is described mainly for malunited calcaneal fractures with considerable loss of height and axial deviation [20,52]; however, AVN of the talus that leads to segmental collapse of the talar dome also may lead to height loss and axial malalignment at the hindfoot after talar fractures. Realignment is achieved similar to malunited calcaneal fractures with a bone block technique [20,52,53]. Reestablishment of talar declination decompresses the ankle joint and relieves tibiotalar impingement secondary to talar collapse [3]. The bone blocks are shaped to correct varus or valgus malalignment of the hindfoot in the coronal plane [2,20]. Correct realignment is checked with intraoperative radiographs after temporary transfixation of the subtalar joint with Kirschner wires. Stable fusion usually is achieved with two 6.5-mm large-fragment screws. Occasionally, subtalar fusion also requires a simultaneous corrective calcaneal osteotomy to correct the hindfoot position [2].

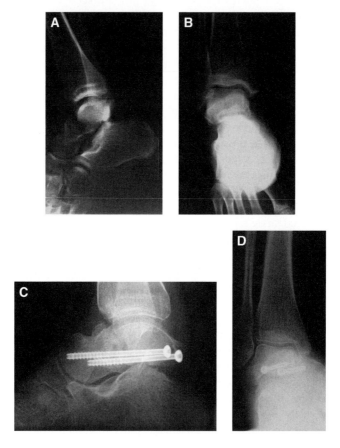

Fig. 3. Type I malunion in a 15-year-old girl who presented 6 months after sustaining a displaced fracture through the anterior talar body (A, B) that had been fixed with screws in persistent subluxation at the subtalar joint (C, D). (E–H) Painful hindfoot deformity with inability to bear weight and severely restricted ankle motion resulted. (I) The ankle joint was affected by a dorsally displaced fragment at the anterior aspect of the talar dome (arrow). The subtalar joint had to be fused with bone block distraction arthrodesis because of a full-thickness cartilage defect, whereas the ankle joint was salvaged by realignment of the talar body. (J, K) 20 months after reconstruction no AVN or arthritic change at the ankle and midtarsal joints was noted. (L, M) Hindfoot alignment was restored with subtle cavus present on both sides. Ankle motion could be restored to near normal (N, O), whereas some eversion and inversion was preserved through the midtarsal joint (P, Q).

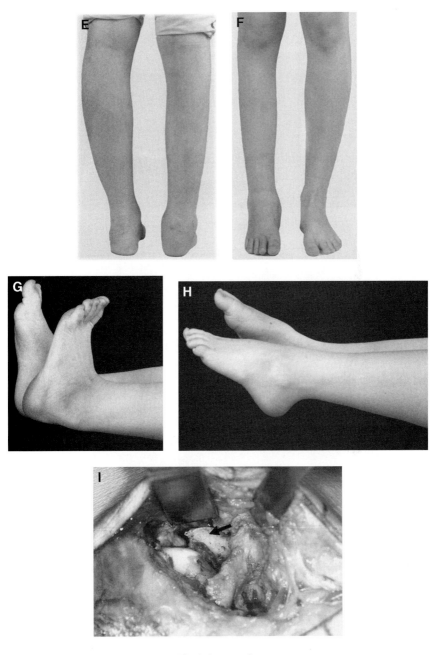

Fig. 3 (*continued*).

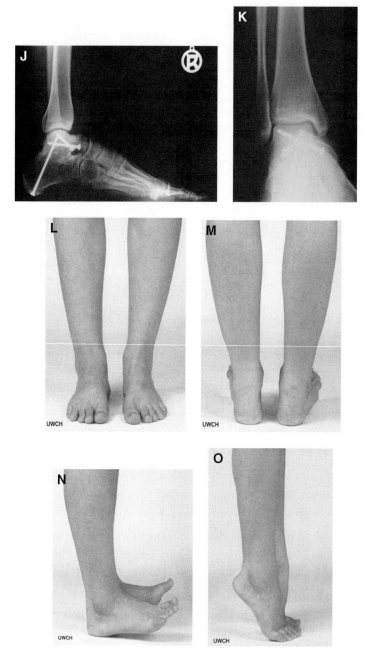

Fig. 3 (*continued*).

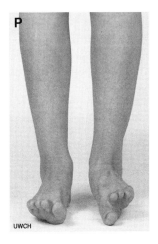 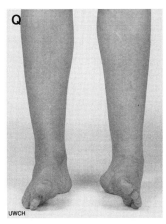

Fig. 3 (*continued*).

Subtalar arthrodesis secondary to talar malunions has not been evaluated separately, and accounts for approximately 10% of all cases in some of the clinical series that dealt predominantly with correction of malunited calcaneal fractures [20,53–55]. In general, subtalar fusion with realignment of the hindfoot provides reliable pain relief with patient satisfaction in 73% to 96% of cases and fusion rates between 86% and 100% [20].

Tibiocalcaneal arthrodesis

With severe collapse of the talus and posttraumatic arthritis of the ankle and subtalar joint and after excision of the talar body secondary to osteomyelitis, tibiocalcaneal arthrodesis remains the only option for salvage (Fig. 4). Like with ankle or subtalar fusion, perfect hindfoot alignment is of absolute importance to achieve a stable, plantigrade foot. Because tibiocalcaneal arthrodesis produces a stiff hindfoot, higher pressures are generated at the midtarsal and tarsometatarsal joints. Any residual malalignment in the sagittal plane (most notably varus deformity) invariably leads to overload of the lateral or medial column, whereas equinus leads to overload of the metatarsals with the development of painful callosities. Nonunion rates increase with the number of fusions performed and the degree of AVN.

Numerous techniques have been described for tibiocalcaneal fusion, including internal fixation with long screws, plates, or a retrograde intramedullary rod and external fixation with a large-pin or small-wire (Ilizarov) frame [18,19,56–59]. The latter also can be used for simultaneous callus distraction to avoid limb-length discrepancy [19,60]. In some cases, a combination of internal and external fixation is used. In the presence of infection (type V malunions), staged reconstruction after aggressive debridement and temporary implantation of local antibiotic beads is recommended [36,61]. In addition, systemic antibiotics are administered for 4 to 6 weeks [61].

The choice of the surgical approach is dictated by the soft tissue conditions, scars from previous surgery, and the planned type of fixation. Anterior midline, medial, lateral, and posterior approaches have been described. To achieve successful fusion, removal of all necrotic and infected bone is mandatory [18,62]. There is no evidence that total talectomy and introduction of a large bone block gives higher fusion rates than does fusion around the remaining body after excision of necrotic tissue [13]. The void that is left after debridement is filled

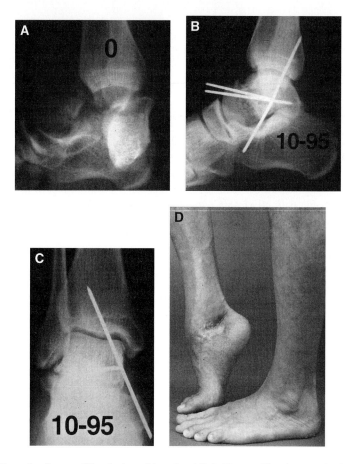

Fig. 4. Example of a type IV malunion of the talus. (*A*) A 37-year-old patient sustained a second-degree open Hawkins type IV fracture–dislocation of his right talus after falling from a height of 3 m. (*B*) After debridement and gross reduction, the fracture was fixed with Kirschner wires. (*C*) The anteroposterior radiograph reveals incomplete reduction of the subtalar joint. After prolonged cast immobilization, the patient was restricted to nonweight bearing for about 1 year. (*D*) He presented to the authors' department 16 months after the injury with a contract equinus deformity and beginning reflex sympathetic dystrophy. Standard radiographs (*E*), CT (*F*), and MRI (*G, H*) show complete AVN of the talar body. (*I*) After excision of all necrotic bone, a large corticocancellous block was used for tibiocalcaneal fusion and was fixed to the viable talar head. (*J, K*) 2 years after the salvage procedure, the patient has a sound fusion and a stable, plantigrade hindfoot.

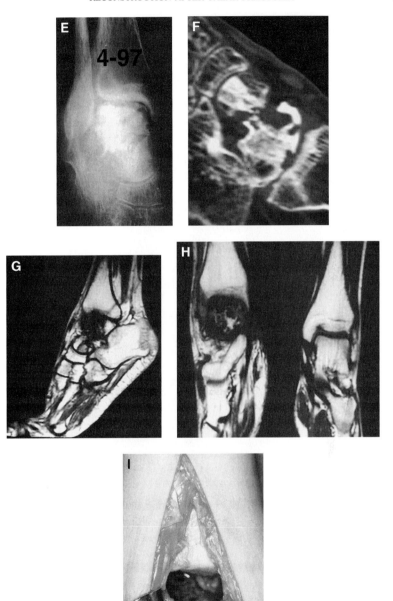

Fig. 4 (*continued*).

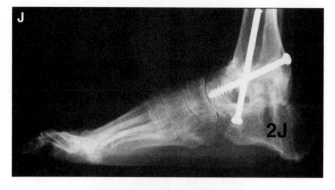

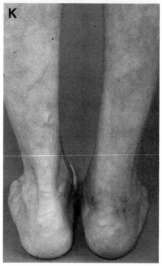

Fig. 4 (*continued*).

with tricortical or cancellous bone graft. Another option is a Blair type of tibio-calcaneal fusion with anterior sliding graft from the tibia to the viable talar head [63]. This approach, practiced in several modifications, reestablishes limb length and continuity, directs forces to the hind- and midfoot, and preserves the essential talonavicular joint [64,65]; however, in the presence of osteomyelitis, total removal of the talar body may be the only option to avoid below-the-knee amputation. After the infection has resolved, bone grafting and tibiocalcaneal fusion are performed as a secondary salvage procedure [19,36]. In active and compliant patients this may be followed by callus distraction to restore limb length; however, patients should be aware of the prolonged course and frequent complications (eg, pin track infections, pin loosening that warrants revision surgery) [19,57,60].

The goals of tibiocalcaneal arthrodesis are reduction of pain and a stable, plantigrade foot. With the fusion of two important joints, a considerable functional impairment prevails. Generally, satisfactory results range between 75% and

87% [56,59,66,67]. Nonunions are seen in 14% of cases [56,66], and infections are seen in less than 10% of cases [18,19,66,67]. Although retrograde nailing seems to provide maximum stability [68], inherent problems after this procedure include stress fracture above the proximal interlocking screws and cortical hypertrophy [59,69].

Again, only a few reports relate exclusively to talar fractures and their sequelae. Gruen and Mears [47] performed arthrodesis of the ankle and subtalar joints with a blade plate for complex nonunions that include segmental bone loss and collapse of the talar body. In the presence of a major soft tissue defect after infection, a microvascular free flap was applied. Three of the 5 patients had excellent results, and 2 patients had good results at a follow-up of 33 months. Gagneux and colleagues [16] obtained solid fusions with intramedullary retrograde nailing in seven of nine cases of complex tibial pilon and talar fractures with severe soft tissue injury. One foot required amputation after failed revascularization, and in one case the nail became unlocked which rendered the fusion unstable. Kitaoka and Patzer [18] performed ankle and subtalar arthrodesis with bone grafting in 16 patients who had osteoarthritis and AVN of the talus. The results were excellent in 5 patients, good in 6 patients, fair in 2 patients, and poor in 3 patients. All 3 patients with a poor result had a nonunion and 2 had malalignment in plantarflexion.

The use of triple arthrodesis for talar malunions and nonunions is reported only anecdotally [5,14,21]. Canale and Kelly [5] found unsatisfactory results after triple arthrodesis for the treatment of varus malalignment of the talar neck. Isolated reports exist on pantalar fusion, which should be a last salvage option for the sequelae of severe talar fractures with complicated courses [56,70].

Some investigators have proposed primary talectomy or fusion for comminuted talar fractures [63,71,72]. The mostly poor results of the few reported cases do not favor this approach [5,10,11,13,73]. Also, early subtalar fusion did not produce earlier revascularization of the talus [5,36,72].

Summary

Residual deformities, malunions, and nonunions of the talus after trauma almost invariably lead to severe disability and pain. Secondary anatomic reconstruction with preservation of the ankle, subtalar, and talonavicular joints may lead to a considerable functional improvement in patients who have minimal AVN of the talus and no symptomatic arthritis. Furthermore, patients should be compliant and free of infection and the cartilage should be viable as determined by MRI and intraoperative assessment. Fusion should be reserved for severe posttraumatic arthritis and should be restricted to the affected joint. Arthrodeses must be combined with correction of the underlying deformity to realign the weight-bearing forces of the foot. Even with complete hindfoot fusion, the talonavicular joint should be preserved whenever possible. Although arthrodeses reportedly provide substantial pain relief, some functional impairment prevails and the long-term outcome is limited by the development of degenerative changes in the adjacent joints. Patients who have severe posttraumatic arthritis and no AVN of the talar dome or gross deformity are amenable for total ankle replacement. This option is especially attractive if the subtalar joint has to be fused.

References

[1] Rammelt S, Winkler J, Heineck J, et al. Anatomical reconstruction of malunited talus fractures. A prospective study of 10 patients followed for 4 years. Acta Orthop 2005;76(4):588–96.

[2] Zwipp H, Rammelt S. Posttraumatic deformity correction at the foot. Zentralbl Chir 2003; 128(3):218–26 [in German].

[3] Sangeorzan BJ, Hansen Jr ST. Early and late posttraumatic foot reconstruction. Clin Orthop Relat Res 1989;(243):86–91.

[4] Hansen ST. Functional reconstruction of the foot and ankle. Philadelphia: Williams & Wilkins; 2000.

[5] Canale ST, Kelly Jr FB. Fractures of the neck of the talus. J Bone Joint Surg Am 1978;60: 143–56.

[6] Lorentzen JE, Christensen SB, Krogsoe O, et al. Fractures of the neck of the talus. Acta Orthop Scand 1977;48(1):115–20.

[7] Peterson L, Goldie IF, Irstam L. Fracture of the neck of the talus. A clinical study. Acta Orthop Scand 1977;48(6):696–706.

[8] Sneppen O, Christensen SB, Krogsoe O, et al. Fracture of the body of the talus. Acta Orthop Scand 1977;48(3):317–24.

[9] Daniels TR, Smith JW, Ross TI. Varus malalignment of the talar neck. Its effect on the position of the foot and on subtalar motion. J Bone Joint Surg Am 1996;78(10):1559–67.

[10] Schuind F, Andrianne Y, Burny F, et al. [Complications following talus trauma]. Aktuelle Traumatol 1985;15(2):82–8 [in German].

[11] Hawkins LG. Fractures of the neck of the talus. J Bone Joint Surg Am 1970;52(5):991–1002.

[12] Parsons SJ. Relation between the occurrence of bony union and outcome for fractures of the lateral process of the talus: a case report and analysis of published reports. Br J Sports Med 2003;37(3):274–6.

[13] Adelaar RS, Madrian JR. Avascular necrosis of the talus. Orthop Clin North Am 2004;35(3): 383–95.

[14] Asencio G, Rebai M, Bertin R, et al. [Pseudarthrosis and non-union of disjunctive talar fractures]. Rev Chir Orthop Reparatrice Appar Mot 2000;86(2):173–80 [in French].

[15] Frawley PA, Hart JA, Young DA. Treatment outcome of major fractures of the talus. Foot Ankle Int 1995;16(6):339–45.

[16] Gagneux E, Gerard F, Garbuio P, et al. [Treatment of complex fractures of the ankle and their sequellae using trans-plantar intramedullary nailing]. Acta Orthop Belg 1997;63(4):294–304 [in French].

[17] Hintermann B, Valderrabano V. Total ankle replacement. Foot Ankle Clin 2003;8(2):375–405.

[18] Kitaoka HB, Patzer GL. Arthrodesis for the treatment of arthrosis of the ankle and osteonecrosis of the talus. J Bone Joint Surg Am 1998;80(3):370–9.

[19] Liener UC, Bauer G, Kinzl L, et al. [Tibiocalcaneal fusion for the treatment of talar necrosis. An analysis of 21 cases]. Unfallchirurg 1999;102(11):848–54 [in German].

[20] Rammelt S, Grass R, Zawadski T, et al. Foot function after subtalar distraction bone-block arthrodesis. A prospective study. J Bone Joint Surg Br 2004;86(5):659–68.

[21] Rockett MS, De Yoe B, Gentile SC, et al. Nonunion of a Hawkin's group II talar neck fracture without avascular necrosis. J Foot Ankle Surg 1998;37(2):156–61.

[22] Zwipp H, Gavlik JM, Rammelt S, et al. Rekonstruktion fehlverheilter Talusfrakturen [Reconstruction of malunited talar fractures]. In: Probst J, Zwipp H, editors. Posttraumatische

Korrektureingriffe nach Fehlheilung an Becken und unterer Extremität Bericht über die 2 Dresdner Unfalltagung am 4 April 1998 [Posttraumatic corrections after malunions at the pelvis and lower extremity]. Sankt Augustin: Hauptverband der gewerblichen Berufsgenossenschaften; 1998. p. 161–80 [in German].

[23] Monroe MT, Manoli II A. Osteotomy for malunion of a talar neck fracture: a case report. Foot Ankle Int 1999;20(3):192–5.

[24] Peterson L, Romanus B, Dahlberg E. Fracture of the collum tali—an experimental study. J Biomech 1976;9(4):277–9.

[25] Sangeorzan BJ, Wagner UA, Harrington RM, et al. Contact characteristics of the subtalar joint: the effect of talar neck misalignment. J Orthop Res 1992;10(4):544–51.

[26] Christensen SB, Lorentzen JE, Krogsoe O, et al. Subtalar dislocation. Acta Orthop Scand 1977;48(6):707–11.

[27] Heckman JD, McLean MR. Fractures of the lateral process of the talus. Clin Orthop 1985; 199:108–13.

[28] Giuffrida AY, Lin SS, Abidi N, et al. Pseudo os trigonum sign: missed posteromedial talar facet fracture. Foot Ankle Int 2003;24(8):642–9.

[29] Cobey JC. Posterior roentgenogram of the foot. Clin Orthop Relat Res 1976;(118):202–7.

[30] Veazey BL, Heckman JD, Galindo MJ, et al. Excision of ununited fractures of the posterior process of the talus: a treatment for chronic posterior ankle pain. Foot Ankle 1992;13(8):453–7.

[31] Mulfinger GL, Trueta J. The blood supply of the talus. J Bone Joint Surg Br 1970;52:160–7.

[32] Mahan KT, Lamy C. Surgical repair of a talar body nonunion. J Am Podiatr Med Assoc 1992; 82(9):454–62.

[33] Migues A, Solari G, Carrasco NM, et al. Repair of talar neck nonunion with indirect corticocancellous graft technique: a case report and review of the literature. Foot Ankle Int 1996; 17(11):690–4.

[34] Moeckel BH, Patterson BM, Inglis AE, et al. Ankle arthrodesis. A comparison of internal and external fixation. Clin Orthop Relat Res 1991;(268):78–83.

[35] Zwipp H, Grass R, Rammelt S, et al. [Arthrodesis - non-union of the ankle. Arthrodesis failed]. Chirurg 1999;70(11):1216–24 [in German].

[36] Rammelt S, Grass R, Brenner P, et al. [Septic necrosis after third-degree open talus fracture in conjunction with complex trauma of the foot (floating talus)]. Trauma Berufskr 2001;3(Suppl 2): 230–5 [in German].

[37] Endres T, Grass R, Rammelt S, et al. Ankle arthrodesis with four cancellous lag screws. Oper Orthop Traumatol 2005;17(4/5):345–60.

[38] Mazur JM, Schwartz E, Simon SR. Ankle arthrodesis. Long-term follow-up with gait analysis. J Bone Joint Surg Am 1979;61(7):964–75.

[39] Morrey BF, Wiedeman Jr GP. Complications and long-term results of ankle arthrodeses following trauma. J Bone Joint Surg Am 1980;62(5):777–84.

[40] Takakura Y, Tanaka Y, Sugimoto K, et al. Long-term results of arthrodesis for osteoarthritis of the ankle. Clin Orthop Relat Res 1999;(361):178–85.

[41] Coester LM, Saltzman CL, Leupold J, et al. Long-term results following ankle arthrodesis for post-traumatic arthritis. J Bone Joint Surg Am 2001;83-A(2):219–28.

[42] Fuchs S, Sandmann C, Skwara A, et al. Quality of life 20 years after arthrodesis of the ankle. A study of adjacent joints. J Bone Joint Surg Br 2003;85(7):994–8.

[43] Morgan CD, Henke JA, Bailey RW, et al. Long-term results of tibiotalar arthrodesis. J Bone Joint Surg Am 1985;67(4):546–50.

[44] Schaap EJ, Huy J, Tonino AJ. Long-term results of arthrodesis of the ankle. Int Orthop 1990; 14(1):9–12.

[45] Ahlberg A, Henricson AS. Late results of ankle fusion. Acta Orthop Scand 1981;52(1):103–5.

[46] Buck P, Morrey BF, Chao EY. The optimum position of arthrodesis of the ankle. A gait study of the knee and ankle. J Bone Joint Surg Am 1987;69(7):1052–62.

[47] Gruen GS, Mears DC. Arthrodesis of the ankle and subtalar joints. Clin Orthop Relat Res 1991;(268):15–20.

[48] Buechel Sr FF, Buechel Jr FF, Pappas MJ. Ten-year evaluation of cementless Buechel-Pappas meniscal bearing total ankle replacement. Foot Ankle Int 2003;24(6):462–72.

[49] Knecht SI, Estin M, Callaghan JJ, et al. The Agility total ankle arthroplasty. Seven to sixteen-year follow-up. J Bone Joint Surg Am 2004;86-A(6):1161–71.

[50] Spirt AA, Assal M, Hansen Jr ST. Complications and failure after total ankle arthroplasty. J Bone Joint Surg Am 2004;86-A(6):1172–8.

[51] Kofoed H. Scandinavian total ankle replacement (STAR). Clin Orthop Relat Res 2004;(424): 73–9.

[52] Carr JB, Hansen ST, Benirschke SK. Subtalar distraction bone block fusion for late complications of os calcis fractures. Foot Ankle 1988;9(2):81–6.

[53] Bednarz PA, Beals TC, Manoli II A. Subtalar distraction bone block fusion: an assessment of outcome. Foot Ankle Int 1997;18(12):785–91.

[54] Dahm DL, Kitaoka HB. Subtalar arthrodesis with internal compression for post-traumatic arthritis. J Bone Joint Surg Br 1998;80(1):134–8.

[55] Easley ME, Trnka HJ, Schon LC, et al. Isolated subtalar arthrodesis. J Bone Joint Surg Am 2000;82(5):613–24.

[56] Papa JA, Myerson MS. Pantalar and tibiotalocalcaneal arthrodesis for post-traumatic osteoarthrosis of the ankle and hindfoot. J Bone Joint Surg Am 1992;74(7):1042–9.

[57] Richter D, Hahn MP, Laun RA, et al. Arthrodesis of the infected ankle and subtalar joint: technique, indications, and results of 45 consecutive cases. J Trauma 1999;47(6):1072–8.

[58] Russotti GM, Johnson KA, Cass JR. Tibiotalocalcaneal arthrodesis for arthritis and deformity of the hind part of the foot. J Bone Joint Surg Am 1988;70(9):1304–7.

[59] Kile TA, Donnelly RE, Gehrke JC, et al. Tibiotalocalcaneal arthrodesis with an intramedullary device. Foot Ankle Int 1994;15(12):669–73.

[60] Hawkins BJ, Langerman RJ, Anger DM, et al. The Ilizarov technique in ankle fusion. Clin Orthop Relat Res 1994;(303):217–25.

[61] Cierny III G, Cook WG, Mader JT. Ankle arthrodesis in the presence of ongoing sepsis. Indications, methods, and results. Orthop Clin North Am 1989;20(4):709–21.

[62] Rzesacz EH, Culemann U, Illgner A, et al. [Homologous talus replacement after talectomy in infection and septic talus necrosis. Experiences with 3 cases]. Unfallchirurg 1997;100(6): 497–501 [in German].

[63] Blair HC. Comminuted fractures and fracture-dislocations of the body of the astragalus. Am J Surg 1943;59:37–43.

[64] Dennis MD, Tullos HS. Blair tibiotalar arthrodesis for injuries to the talus. J Bone Joint Surg Am 1980;62(1):103–7.

[65] Van Bergeyk A, Stotler W, Beals T, et al. Functional outcome after modified Blair tibiotalar arthrodesis for talar osteonecrosis. Foot Ankle Int 2003;24(10):765–70.

[66] Chou LB, Mann RA, Yaszay B, et al. Tibiotalocalcaneal arthrodesis. Foot Ankle Int 2000; 21(10):804–8.

[67] Moore TJ, Prince R, Pochatko D, Smith JW, Fleming S. Retrograde intramedullary nailing for ankle arthrodesis. Foot Ankle Int 1995;16(7):433–6.

[68] Berend ME, Glisson RR, Nunley JA. A biomechanical comparison of intramedullary nail and crossed lag screw fixation for tibiotalocalcaneal arthrodesis. Foot Ankle Int 1997;18(10): 639–43.

[69] Thordarson DB, Chang D. Stress fractures and tibial cortical hypertrophy after tibiotalocalcaneal arthrodesis with an intramedullary nail. Foot Ankle Int 1999;20(8):497–500.

[70] Weber M, Schwer H, Zilkens KW, et al. Tibio-calcaneo-naviculo-cuboidale arthrodesis: 6 patients followed for 1–8 years. Acta Orthop Scand 2002;73(1):98–103.

[71] Coltart WD. Aviator's astragalus. J Bone Jont Surg Br 1952;34:546–66.

[72] Hantira H, Al Sayed H, Barghash I. Primary ankle fusion using Blair technique for severely comminuted fracture of the talus. Med Princ Pract 2003;12(1):47–50.

[73] Pennal GF. Fractures of the talus. Clin Orthop 1963;30:53–63.

ELSEVIER
SAUNDERS

Foot Ankle Clin N Am
11 (2006) 85–103

FOOT AND
ANKLE CLINICS

Post–Calcaneus Fracture Reconstruction

Florian Nickisch, MD, Robert B. Anderson, MD*

OrthoCarolina, PA, 1001 Blythe Boulevard, Suite 200, Charlotte, NC 28203, USA

This article outlines the pathoanatomy of malunited calcaneal fractures and reviews the literature on resulting painful sequelae, diagnostic work-up, as well as reconstructive treatment options and their outcome.

The calcaneus is the most commonly fractured tarsal bone, and accounts for approximately 60% to 70% of tarsal fractures and 2% of all fractures [1]. Most calcaneal fractures are intra-articular (56–75%) [1,2]. They affect a young and active population and have great impact on the work force and society. In 1916, Cotton and Henderson [3] wrote that "the man who breaks his heel bone is done, so far as his industrial future is concerned" and in 1942, Bankart [4] stated that "the results of treatment of crush fractures of the os calcis are rotten." Numerous operative and nonoperative treatment regimens have been proposed.

Based on the early experiences of Bohler [5] and Letournel [6], Benirschke [7] and Sanders and colleagues [8] developed open reduction and internal fixation (ORIF) through an extensile lateral approach. This technique seems to lead to more favorable results [7,9–11] compared with conservative treatment. In a recent prospective randomized multicenter study, Buckley [10] noted that female patients, patients who had displaced calcaneal fractures, and non workers compensation patients benefited from ORIF. There is a considerable learning curve. To avoid the soft tissue complications that are associated with ORIF, several percutaneous and minimally invasive reduction techniques have been developed

---

* Corresponding author.
E-mail address: drrba@carolina.rr.com (R.B. Anderson).

Box 1. Painful late sequelae of malunited calcaneus fractures

Subtalar arthritis
Calcaneocuboid arthritis
Heel widening (shoe wear problems)
Peroneal impingement and calcaneofibular abutment
Loss of hindfoot height (shoe wear problems)
Anterior ankle impingement
Decreased midfoot motion with development of osteoarthritis
    in adjacent joints
Hindfoot malalignment (varus more common than valgus)
Flattening of the longitudinal arch
Talonavicular subluxation
Unrecognized compartment syndrome
Nerve problems (sural more common than tibial)
Chronic pain syndromes
Smashed heel syndrome
First metatarso-phalangeal stiffness secondary to flexor hallucis
    longus entrapment
Haglund's deformity secondary to malunited tongue fragment
Forefoot malalignment

---

for selected fracture patterns [12–16]. Calcaneus fractures are disabling injuries that are associated with long-term complications (Box 1).

Pathoanatomy and late complications

Calcaneus fractures typically result from axial load, as in falls from a height or from motor vehicle accidents. Because the mechanical axis falls medial to the tuberosity, the lateral process of the talus shears the tuberosity from the remainder of the calcaneal body at the "critical angle of Gissane." This creates the primary fracture line that divides the calcaneus into anteromedial and posterolateral (tuberosity) fragments. The sustentaculum tali (as part of the anteromedial fragment) usually remains attached to the talar body, tethered by the strong interosseous and medial ligaments. The tuberosity fragment displaces superiorly and laterally, and into varus, which results in a shortened and flattened calcaneus with loss of hindfoot height (decreased Böhler's angle). The talus assumes a more horizontal, dorsiflexed position with a radiographic decreased talar declination angle (Fig. 1). This leads to painful anterior impingement of the talar neck on the anterior tibial plafond (Fig. 2). The trapezoidal talar body (wider anterior dimension) wedges in the ankle mortise, which diminishes dorsiflexion and rotational and translational movements of the ankle joint. This may accelerate

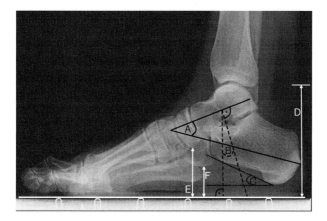

Fig. 1. Weight-bearing lateral radiograph of a normal foot demonstrating radiographic measurements for hindfoot alignment. A, talocalcaneal angle; B, talar declination angle; C, calcaneal pitch angle; D, talo-calcaneal height; E, navicular to floor distance; F, cuboid to floor distance. (*Adapted from* Buch BD, Myerson MS, Miller SD. Primary subtalar arthrodesis for the treatment of comminuted calcaneal fractures. Foot Ankle Int 1996;17(2):64; with permission.) © 1996 by the American Orthopaedic Foot and Ankle Society.

development of ankle arthritis [17,18]. Loss of hindfoot height may pose significant problems with shoe wear, because the malleoli contact the shoe counter, and cause limb length discrepancy. The decreased calcaneal body height and length shorten the lever arm of the gastroc–soleus complex, and thus, decreases push-off power.

Because of the coupled motion of the subtalar and transverse tarsal joints, the varus hindfoot locks Chopart's joint and thus stiffens the foot [19]. The talonavicular joint is unable to unlock during gait and prevent shock absorption. This places unphysiologic, high loads on the adjacent articulations, and can lead to accelerated breakdown of these joints. Gait analysis demonstrates lateralization of the center of pressure progression and increased pressure under the head of the

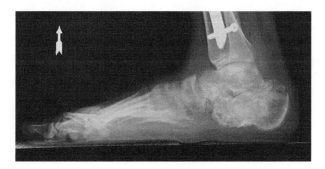

Fig. 2. Calcaneus fracture malunion in an 18-year-old man 6 months after he sustained multitrauma. Note the significant incongruity of the subtalar joint, loss of talocalcaneal height, negative Böhler's angle, calcaneal shortening, horizontal talus with talonavicular subluxation, and anterior ankle impingement.

fifth metatarsal, if any displacement exists [20,21]. This may be due to heel varus or loss of subtalar joint motion. Varus displacement of the heel leads to eccentric loading of the ankle and knee joints, which causes increased loads on the medial side and attenuation of the lateral structures [22,23]. Occasionally, valgus displacement of the tuberosity occurs.

As the talus is impacted further into the calcaneal body, the calcaneal wall is displaced laterally. This lateral wall "blow-out" and lateral displacement of the tuberosity is responsible for the heel widening (Fig. 3). This diminishes the available space for the lateral structures (peroneal tendons, sural nerve). Peroneal impingement, tendonitis, or tears of the tendons have been described, and can be a source of chronic pain. In extreme cases, painful calcaneofibular abutment may occur (see Fig. 3C) [24]. Dislocation of the peroneal tendons occurs after high-energy injuries with severe calcaneal displacement. With appropriate surgical reduction of the fracture, the tendons return to their anatomic position. Chronically dislocated tendons can be a source of ongoing pain and disability. The sural nerve can be injured from traction or impingement that results in neuritis or neuroma formation [22]. The medial and lateral plantar nerves are at risk with severe valgus displacement, lateral fracture dislocations, or medial bony impingement.

The primary fracture traverses the posterior articular facet of the calcaneus. Depending on the amount and direction of the absorbed energy, "secondary fracture lines" propagate in anterior and posterior directions from the primary fracture line. This leads to comminution of the posterior facet and the anterior process. Therefore, posttraumatic arthritis of the subtalar joint is seen commonly after displaced intra-articular calcaneus fractures. Anatomic reduction of the posterior articular facet reduces the incidence of posttraumatic osteoarthritis [22]. Significantly altered contact pressures occur with intra-articular step-offs as small as 1 mm [13,25]. In a prospective randomized study, patients who were treated nonoperatively were five times more likely to require late subtalar arthrodesis.

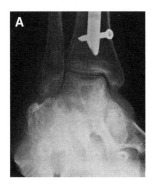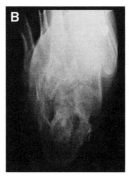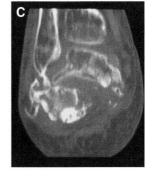

Fig. 3. (A, B) Weight-bearing mortise view and axial view of the same patient as in Fig. 2 demonstrate significant lateral wall blow out with heel widening and calcaneofibular abutment. (C) Coronal CT image of malunited calcaneal fracture dislocation with calcaneofibular abutment and dislocated peroneal tendons.

Other risk factors for late subtalar fusion included male gender, workers compensation, heavy labor, fracture patterns with a Böhler's angle less than 0°, as well as Sanders type IV fractures [26]. The patients who sustain high-energy injuries may develop posttraumatic arthritis, despite anatomic reduction [8], because of cartilage damage. Irreversible damage was demonstrated to occur to the articular cartilage after a single, high-energy impact load [27]. A primary subtalar arthrodesis may be beneficial for severely comminuted fractures (Sanders type IV) [8,28,29]. Not all patients with radiographic evidence of posttraumatic subtalar arthritis are symptomatic [30,31].

As many as 50% of calcaneus fractures involve the calcaneocuboid (CC) articulation; an anterolateral fragment of the calcaneus displaces through the joint in an anterior–lateral–superior direction. This displaced fragment can block motion at the CC joint [8]. Posttraumatic arthritis or deformity of the CC joint is common on radiographs but frequently is asymptomatic. Patients who have this type of deformity or arthritis should be evaluated carefully before fusing this joint [31–33].

Compartment syndrome of the foot can occur after calcaneal fracture. Clawing of the lesser toes, and sensory disturbances in the medial or lateral plantar nerves may be encountered if this is not treated [34]. The calcaneal compartment of the foot contains the quadratus plantae muscle and the posterior tibial neurovascular bundle (lateral and plantar medial nerves more distally) on the plantar surface of the foot [35]. Sequelae of deep posterior compartment syndrome include contracture and scarring of the posterior tibial muscle, the flexor hallucis longus, and the flexor digitorum longus, and results in a fixed cavovarus deformity. The incidence of compartment syndrome of the foot associated with calcaneus fractures is 4.7% to 17% [36].

A superolateral exostosis from a malunited tongue-type fracture can irritate the Achilles tendon, much like a Haglund's deformity [37]. Painful plantar exostosis usually is seen after nonoperative treatment or inadequately reduced high-energy calcaneal fractures that involve the plantar cortex [3,8]. Other causes of ongoing pain include nerve entrapment, complex regional pain syndrome, and smashed heel pad syndrome [8,29].

Diagnostic work-up

Clinical evaluation

The soft tissue envelope has to be examined carefully for previous open injuries and old incisions because this may influence the surgical approach. Uneven shoe wear and plantar callosities indicate uneven weight distribution. Alignment of the ankle, hindfoot, and forefoot (varus/valgus/cavus/planus) in stance and gait are recorded. Active and passive range of motion of all joints are assessed, including passive correctability of deformity.

Lateral pain may be caused by peroneal tendon pathology, subtalar arthritis, CC arthritis, hardware, or sural nerve problems. The peroneal tendons are palpated along their entire course and their anatomic location is verified. Resisted eversion may aggravate symptoms. Loss of active eversion may be due to dislocated, scarred, or torn peroneal tendons. Motion may be blocked by lateral impingement, posttraumatic hindfoot stiffness, or severe subtalar arthritis. Typically, subtalar arthritis pain is worse with ambulation on uneven ground, and is reproduced by passive hindfoot inversion and eversion. Pain at rest, which is associated with paresthesias or numbness on the lateral side of the foot, should raise suspicion for problems that are related to the sural nerve or chronic regional pain syndrome (CRPS). These patients may be unable to tolerate wearing high-top shoes or tight socks, because of pressure on the nerve. There may be a positive Tinel's sign. Diagnostic injections of the subtalar joint, CC joint, peroneal sheath, or the sural nerve with a local anesthetic (1% lidocaine, 0.5% bupivacaine) may differentiate these sources of pain. Myerson and Quill [29] found that these blocks were helpful in 87.5% of their patients. We recommend fluoroscopic guidance and injection of radio-opaque dye to ensure correct needle placement [38].

Anterior pain may be caused by talar neck impingement or scar tissue in the ankle. Typically, impingement symptoms are reproduced by forced dorsiflexion of the ankle. Arthritis in the tibiotalar and talonavicular joints may cause anterior ankle pain. Careful clinical examination and selective diagnostic injections of the tibiotalar or talonavicular joint establish the correct diagnosis and predict the success of surgical treatment.

Plantar pain can be secondary to plantar exostosis that is identified readily on plain radiographs. Smashed heel pad syndrome results in a diffusely tender heel pad. Atrophy of the heel may occur.

Poorly localized pain should raise suspicion for nerve-related problems or CRPS. If symptoms are mostly medial and plantar, then posttraumatic tarsal tunnel syndrome should be considered. These patients may complain of pain, sensory changes, or paresthesias in a tibial nerve distribution. Tenderness over the course of the tibial nerve or radiation to the plantar aspect of the heel or the sole of the foot, as well as a positive Tinel's sign, may be present. Symptoms may be exacerbated by dorsiflexion of the foot and ankle [39]. Weakness of the intrinsic musculature secondary to a nerve injury is clinically similar to a missed compartment syndrome. Electrophysiologic testing can establish a diagnosis. Trophic skin changes can be present. CRPS should be ruled out by lumbar sympathetic blocks [36].

Radiographic evaluation

Standard radiographs include weight-bearing lateral and anteroposterior views of the foot, and a posterior tangential view of the calcaneus (Harris view). Radiographs of the normal foot demonstrate normal alignment and radiographic measurements. Anteroposterior and mortise views of the ankle are added if ankle pathology is suspected. Plain radiographs are useful to evaluate the severity of arthritis (ankle, subtalar joint, transverse tarsal joint), gross alignment, and existing deformities. The Harris view and anteroposterior or mortise views of the ankle can demonstrate heel widening and calcaneofibular impingement (see Fig. 3A, B). The radiographic findings do not necessarily correlate with clinical symptoms [31]. A multitude of radiographic measurements, such as hindfoot height, Böhler's angle, lateral talocalcaneal angle, calcaneal inclination angle, and talar declination angle, have been used for the evaluation of calcaneus fractures and malunions (see Fig. 1) [28,29,40,41]. A Böhler's angle of less than 0° and Sanders type IV fracture pattern are highly predictive for late subtalar fusion [26,42]. Myerson and Quill [29] used a loss of hindfoot height of more than 8 mm, compared with the contralateral foot, and a talar declination angle of less than 20° as an indication for distraction bone block arthrodesis. Huang and colleagues [43] adopted these criteria to decide whether to perform an in situ subtalar arthrodesis or a subtalar arthrodesis with plantar sliding calcaneal osteotomy. In 2003, Zwipp and Rammelt [15] proposed a classification system for calcaneal malunions to guide their surgical treatment (Box 2). They recommend computer-assisted three-dimensional preoperative planning for more severe deformities (types 3–5). Conversely, Chandler and colleagues [33] and Flemister and colleagues [44] found no correlation between functional outcome (assessed by the American Orthopedic Foot and Ankle Society [AOFAS] hindfoot score) and hindfoot height or talar declination angle. Radiographic measurements may assist in preoperative planning, but should not be relied upon for surgical decision making.

CT provides more detailed information on the degree of arthritis and the three-dimensional deformity. The peroneal tendons are visualized and possible dislocation detected [45]. Stephens and Sanders [32] devised a validated treatment algorithm for calcaneal malunions based on a CT classification system (Fig.4) [46]. This classification system is based solely on nonweight-bearing coronal CT images, and does not address the loss of hindfoot height, or talar

---

Box 2. Zwipp classification of calcaneal malunions

Type 1: subtalar incongruence
Type 2: plus hindfoot varus/valgus
Type 3: plus loss of height
Type 4: plus translation
Type 5: plus talar tilt

From Zwipp H, Rammelt S. Posttraumatic deformity correction at the foot. Zentralbl Chir 2003;128(3):221.

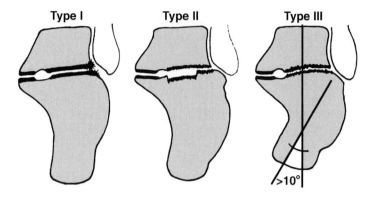

Fig. 4. Stephens CT classification for calcaneal malunions. Type I: large lateral wall exostosis with no or minimal lateral subtalar arthrosis and no malalignment. Type II: lateral wall exostosis, significant subtalar arthrosis, and malalignment (varus) less than 10°. Type III: lateral wall exostosis, significant subtalar arthrosis and malalignment (varus) greater than 10°. (*Adapted from* Stephens H, Sanders R. Calcaneal malunions: results of prognostic computed tomography classification system. Foot Ankle Int 1996;17(7):396; with permission.) © 1996 by the American Orthopaedic Foot and Ankle Society.

declination. Indications for distraction bone block arthrodesis or corrective osteotomies must be determined by using standing radiographs.

Treatment

Conservative treatment

Pain and function may improve for at least 12 months after severe ankle and hindfoot injuries [1]. Thus, conservative treatment (eg, activity modification, shoewear modification, orthotics, medical pain control, rest, ice, compression, and elevation protocol) should be offered initially. Gross deformity with significant lateral impingement in young, active patients may be an indication for earlier surgical intervention [47]. Revascularization of devascularized bone and soft tissues can occur during this time. Some of the late problems after calcaneal fractures (eg, CRPS, smashed heel pad syndrome) may be made worse by surgical intervention. Older age, less education, workers compensation status, smoking, and preexisting comorbidity have a negative effect on surgical intervention [10,46]. A double upright brace or a custom-made Arizona-type brace may reduce symptoms in patients who have subtalar arthritis. [48]

Surgical treatment

Surgical treatment of calcaneal malunions should address all of the pathology and re-establish normal hindfoot anatomy. Depending on the patient's complaints and the severity of the deformity, more limited surgical procedures may be appropriate.

Lateral decompression

In the early twentieth century, Cotton [3] used a Kocher-type curvilinear, lateral incision to perform lateral decompression. Old incisions from a previous open reduction should be used. The lateral calcaneal wall is dissected sub-periosteally, and is excised generously with an osteotome. Pathology of the peroneal tendons or the sural nerve may be addressed at the same time. Braly and colleagues [49] reported on 11 patients who underwent lateral calcaneal exostectomy combined with proximal neurolysis of the sural nerve or excision of sural neuromas. Peroneal tenolysis was performed and dislocated tendons were z-lengthened and relocated; these were followed by repair or reconstruction of the peroneal retinaculum. They reported a success rate of 46%. Z-lengthening of the peroneal tendons is only necessary in cases of severe contracture [48]. Lateral decompression is recommended for Stephens type I malunions with a large lateral exostosis, and minimal arthritis of the subtalar and CC joints without significant deformity [32]. If lateral subtalar arthritis is present, this portion of the joint is included in the exostectomy. The lateral wall resection can be extended anteriorly to include the lateral 25% of the anterior process of the calcaneus, because this portion of the CC joint often is arthritic [46]. This frees up the transverse tarsal joint which is blocked by the malunited anterolateral fracture fragment, and corrects forefoot varus or valgus in flexible deformities [46]. An extensile lateral approach allows direct inspection of the peroneal tendons. Dislocated peroneal tendons often fall back into their usual anatomic location after adequate lateral decompression. If the superior extensor retinaculum needs to be repaired, a separate incision is used. Range of motion exercises should be started as soon as possible to prevent hindfoot and ankle stiffness. Repair of the peroneal tendons or retinaculum has to be protected postoperatively. The average postoperative AOFAS hindfoot score of the five Stephens type I malunions that were treated in Clare and colleagues' [46] series was 68.2 at a minimum follow-up of 2 years. Stephens and Sanders [32] reported six excellent results and one good result; 50% of their patients had improved range of motion.

In situ subtalar arthrodesis

In situ subtalar arthrodesis, which is performed without an attempt to increase calcaneal height, is recommended for calcaneal malunions with minimal deformity and significant subtalar arthritis (Stephens type II, Zwipp type 1) [15,29, 32,46]; it can be combined with lateral decompression if symptoms of lateral impingement are present. Patients who are at risk for wound healing complications or bony nonunion, who otherwise would be candidates for distraction subtalar fusion, may be candidates for an in situ fusion.

The patient is positioned supine with a bump under the ipsilateral hip if a modified Ollier or horizontal sinus tarsi approach is used. In patients who had a previous ORIF, lateral positioning allows use of the previous incision [15,33,44,51–54]. After distraction of the joint with a bone spreader or joint distractor, the articular surfaces of all facets of the subtalar joint are denuded to subchondral bone with osteotomes, curettes, or burrs. All sclerotic and avascular bone must be removed because this influences union rates [53]. If visualization remains difficult after joint distraction, a portion of the lateral process of the talus can be excised [50]. In cases with mild fixed preoperative varus or valgus deformity, additional bone can be removed from the lateral or medial side of the posterior facet [51]. Multiple perforations in the subchondral bone are created with a small drill or K-wire to facilitate revascularization and fusion. Fish-scaling of the subchondral bone and the tarsal canal with an osteotome may increase the chance of bone union [51,53]. Preservation of the soft tissue under the talar neck and the interosseous ligament protects the bone blood supply [22]. After irrigation of the joint and debris removal, the fusion site is bone grafted with local autograft from the resected bone. Alternatively, tibial or iliac crest autograft or cancellous allograft may be used. The guide pins for cannulated screws can be placed from the posteroinferior aspect of the heel to the desired point on the superior surface of the calcaneus, perpendicular to the posterior facet. An anterior cruciate drill guide can facilitate correct pin placement [51]. The subtalar joint is reduced with the heel in approximately 5° of valgus, and the guide pins are advanced into the talus under fluoroscopic control. If solid, large fragment screws are used, reduction can be held temporarily with K-wires or Steinmann pins.

Two partially threaded large fragment (6.5 mm, 7.0 mm, 7.3 mm, 8.0 mm) screws are placed percutaneously, from the posteroplantar aspect of the calcaneal tuberosity, just superior to the weight-bearing surface. To achieve maximum stability, they are placed into the talar body, perpendicular to the posterior facet, in a slightly divergent fashion [44,46,47,53]. In cases with a low talar declination angle (horizontal talus), one of the screws is placed more anteriorly into the talar neck to pull the talus into a more normal, plantarflexed position. This also can be achieved with a screw from the plantar-lateral margin of the anterior process of the calcaneus into talar neck or head. Violation of the talonavicular joint is a risk [46]. Alternatively, screws may be placed through a second incision from the superolateral talar shoulder, or from the anterior talar neck into the calcaneal body [47]. The latter bears a certain risk of injury to the dorsal neurovascular bundle, and may lead to impingement of the screw head on the anterior tibia with ankle dorsiflexion. Mann and colleagues used a single 7.0-mm lagged cancellous screw [51]. Using this technique, Haskell and colleagues [54] reported a fusion rate of 98% in a series of 101 arthrodeses. Newer implants, like the ideal compression screw (I.C.O.S., Newdeal Inc., Vienne, France), may allow a greater degree of joint compression [55].

This dense bone should be predrilled to avoid fractures. Fluoroscopic orthogonal views of the ankle and foot verify correct screw placement. Additional bone graft is packed into any exposed spaces of the subtalar joint, and the wound is closed in layers. Postoperatively, patients are placed in a short-leg posterior splint in neutral position until the wounds are healed (typically 2 weeks). A short-leg cast or removable boot with a rocker sole is applied. Weight bearing is restricted for 6 to 8 weeks, and then is advanced as tolerated with a walking boot or short-leg cast. Usually, radiographic union is observed after 10 to 14 weeks. Patients are encouraged to wear well-cushioned, accommodating shoes and to refrain from high-impact activities to minimize stresses on the adjacent joints.

Most published series report good results after in situ subtalar fusion, with union rates greater than 90%; high rates of patient satisfaction; significant improvement of pain and function, as demonstrated by objective outcome measures (AOFAS score); and low complication rates [29,44,46,51,52]. Nevertheless, foot function is far from normal—even in the best of scenarios—with modified AOFAS scores (maximum score of 94) in the 70s [29,33,44,46,52]. Most patients have difficulty walking on uneven ground and prefer lace-up walking shoes without heels. In the largest published series (143 patients/152 feet), Easley and colleagues [53] pointed out several problems. The overall union rate was 84% (combined in situ and distraction bone block arthrodesis). Risk factors for nonunion include a history of smoking (72% union compared with 92% in nonsmokers), avascular areas of bone at the subtalar joint (62% union), and revision surgery (71% union). There was no significant relationship between clinical outcome or union rate and the pathologic findings that led to subtalar fusion. A trend toward worse results with posttraumatic etiologies was noted [53]. Other complications included infection, prominent hardware, symptomatic malalignment, lateral impingement, and problems related to the sural nerve. Chandler and colleagues [33] reported significantly lower AOFAS scores in patients who had these problems.

Distraction bone block arthrodesis

Distraction bone block arthrodesis [39,47] of the subtalar joint is indicated for calcaneal malunions with subtalar arthritis, significant loss of hindfoot height, and symptomatic anterior ankle impingement that is caused by a horizontal talus (Zwipp type 3). Radiographically, this is determined by a low talar declination angle, and possibly, degenerative changes in the ankle joint with anterior osteophytes (see Fig. 2) [33,44]. Chandler and colleagues [33] recommended distraction arthrodesis for patients who had disabling ankle pain that was reproduced by forced dorsiflexion and ankle dorsiflexion of less than 10°. A concomitant osteotomy may correct major varus or valgus malalignment [47].

Preoperative evaluation establishes an intra-articular origin for pain, likely traumatic arthritis, and the diagnosis can be confirmed with selective injections of the subtalar joint. In addition, the patient may complain of anterior ankle pain, secondary to a loss of normal talar declination angle. Preoperative CT imaging assesses for lateral wall widening; soft tissue window techniques also may assess for peroneal tendon pathology (ie, dislocation).

The ideal patient should have no associated medical problems, and should have good vascularity and skin condition. Smokers should be advised to have surgery after stopping nicotine use because of an increased risk of infection, nonunion, and wound-healing problems.

A popliteal block, combined with general anesthetic, is used for anesthesia. The popliteal block assists postoperative pain control. The patient is positioned in the lateral decubitus or prone position. A thigh tourniquet is applied, and the leg and posterior iliac crest are prepped and draped, if needed. A 5- to 10-cm longitudinal posterolateral incision (Gallie) is made just lateral to the Achilles tendon [56]. Care should be taken to avoid injury to the sural nerve and lesser saphenous vein in the proximal portion of the incision. In patients who have sural nerve symptoms, the nerve can be excised and buried in the soft tissues. Some investigators recommend a modified Kocher incision [57], whereas others recommend the extensile lateral approach, especially for patients with retained hardware from previous ORIF [17,46]; however this may lead to a higher rate of wound complications in the horizontal limb of the incision, because tension-free closure may be difficult after distraction of the subtalar joint and reconstitution of a more normal hindfoot height [40].

After the deep crural fascia is incised, the interval between the flexor hallucis longus and the peroneus longus tendons is used for access to the subtalar joint.

Many of the patients will have retained hardware over the lateral aspect of the calcaneus. These screws can be removed percutaneously, using fluoroscopic imaging. A small incision can be made over the sinus tarsi to assist with screw and plate removal. The plate itself is removed by way of the posterolateral incision, by sliding it out in a posterior direction after the screws are removed. A lateral wall decompression can be performed for cases with bone extending into the subfibular region. A 0.5-inch to 0.75-inch osteotome is directed from posterior to anterior and exits just short of the CC joint. This bone can be used for local bone grafting.

The posterior aspects of the tibio-talar and subtalar joints are now exposed. Usually, the talus is displaced into the body of the calcaneus. Care must be taken not to violate the articular surface of the tibio-talar joint. A Hintermann retractor is applied to the medial aspect with pins placed percutaneously into the calcaneus and talus. This prevents varus malalignment with distraction applied. The tendo-Achilles may be contracted significantly which makes distraction difficult. A gastrocnemius recession by way of a separate incision on the posteromedial aspect of the mid-calf may correct this. With distraction applied, the degenerated subtalar joint surfaces are visualized and prepared for arthrodesis. Remaining articular surfaces of the posterior and medial facets are removed at a subchondral level. If distraction is hindered by contracted and scarred medial structures, an angled curette or periosteal elevator can be used for blunt subperiosteal release of these tissues off the medial calcaneal wall. Care must be taken to prevent injury to the posteromedial neurovascular bundle.

Fluoroscopic lateral radiographs help to determine the proper amount of distraction, based on the talar declination. An appropriately sized interposition bone graft is fashioned. The use of two separate grafts, placed side by side, is beneficial if varus/valgus alignment needs to be corrected (Zwipp type 2 malunion) [15]. If a single bone block is used, it should be placed slightly medial to prevent varus malalignment [47]. Clare and colleagues [46] used the previously excised lateral wall fragment for distraction. The authors prefer allograft for larger corrections. Iliac crest wedges are selected for height restoration of 1 cm or less; femoral head allografts are used for cases that require more correction. The graft is made into a trapezoid shape, while maintaining the cortex along the posterior aspect. The lateral aspect of the wedge is made slightly shorter than the medial aspect to ensure that varus malalignment is avoided. The wedge is inserted, together with local bone graft to fill any small defects. Distraction is released, and additional cancellous graft is packed into the remaining spaces.

In cases of more severe deformity, which is expressed by a negative Böhler's angle, Zwipp and colleagues recommend an additional, plantar-based closing wedge osteotomy of the calcaneal tuberosity [15].

Fixation of the subtalar joint is accomplished with the use of 6.5- to 7.3-mm cannulated screws. Despite the theoretic advantage of fully threaded screws to prevent graft collapse and recurrent deformity, the use of partially threaded screws—placed in a variety of configurations—is well described [53,58,59]. Two screws are placed percutaneously through stab incisions from the posteroinferior aspect of the calcaneal tuberosity into the talar dome [40]. The first screw is placed anterior, entering from the plantar aspect of the calcaneus and extending into the talar neck, compressing across the anterior subtalar joint. The second screw is placed posterior, from the plantar aspect (Fig. 5). This screw is fully threaded to help prevent collapse of the graft. Fluoroscopic imaging in lateral and axial planes ensures proper screw placement. Anteroposterior and mortise views of the ankle should be checked to assure that none of the screws violates the ankle joint.

All wounds are closed in layers. A plaster splint is applied and is converted to a cast when swelling allows. The patient is kept strictly nonweight bearing for 6 to 8 weeks, depending upon the quality of the bone and other healing factors. A short-leg walking cast is used for 4 to 6 weeks, which is followed by a walker boot for a similar period of time. Physical therapy can be instituted to

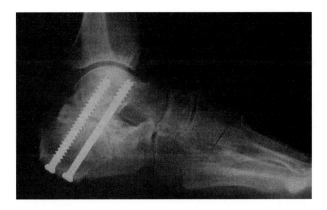

Fig. 5. The authors' technique for subtalar distraction bone block arthrodesis with structural allograft.

assist with edema control, desensitization, gait training, range of motion, and strengthening exercises.

The clinical results of subtalar distraction bone block arthrodesis are comparable to those of in situ subtalar fusion. Most reported series show significant improvement of pain and function with AOFAS scores between 69 and 75 (compared with 20–40 preoperatively), and satisfactory restoration of talocalcaneal height [16,41,44,57–60]. With the use of tricortical iliac crest bone graft, the reported nonunion rate is between 0% and 14% [40,41,59,60]. Besides smoking, which increased the risk of nonunion significantly [41,53,61], factors that are associated with nonunion include revision surgery, areas of avascular bone at the fusion site, and possibly, the use of structural allograft. The nonunion rate with structural allograft may be higher than autograft and may reach rates of 40% [53]. Other complications of this procedure include dislocation of the bone block, malunion (most commonly varus), pain from prominent hardware, infection, and sural and medial plantar nerve problems (neuritis, neuroma, neuralgia) [40,41,53,57,59,60]. Problems that were related to the iliac crest bone graft donor site did not exceed 6% in any of the published series [40,59,60].

Vertical sliding corrective osteotomy with subtalar fusion

Popularized by Huang and colleagues [43], this procedure (Fig. 6) offers an alternative to distraction bone block arthrodesis for patients with difficulty with impingement of the malleoli on the shoe counter because of loss of height. Caution has to be exercised when using this procedure on patients who have anterior ankle impingement, because correction of the talar declination angle and decompression of the anterior ankle joint are minimal.

The patient is placed in a lateral decubitus position. In its original description, an extensile lateral approach was used. A slightly oblique, vertical incision, just posterior to the posterior facet of the subtalar joint as proposed by Hansen [47], may be safer to avoid wound complications. The sural nerve has to be protected. In patients who have lateral impingement symptoms, a lateral wall exostectomy can be performed. The calcaneal tuberosity is osteotomized vertically—just posterior to the articular surface—with an oscillating saw. To avoid injury to the medial neurovascular structures, the osteotomy is completed with an osteotome through the medial calcaneal wall. The tuberosity fragment is shifted plantarward. Lengthening of the Achilles tendon may be necessary to achieve the desired plantar translation. The subtalar joint is debrided and packed with autogenous graft from the excised lateral wall. Large fragment screws are placed perpendicular to the osteotomy and the subtalar joint.

The literature on this technique is scarce. Seven of the twelve patients in Huang and colleagues' [43] series were satisfied completely with the outcome; however, no objective, universal outcome tool was used.

Procedures to correct severe deformity

To correct severe deformities (Stephens type III, Zwipp types 4 and 5) that result from high-energy injuries, correction in three planes may be necessary.

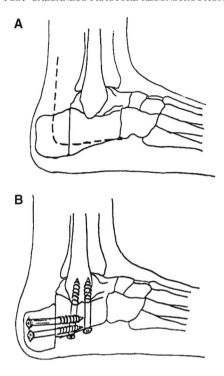

Fig. 6. (*A–B*) Vertical sliding calcaneal osteotomy with subtalar arthrodesis. (*From* Huang P, Fu Y, Cheng Y, et al. Subtalar arthrodesis for late sequelae of calcaneal fractures: fusion in situ versus fusion with sliding corrective osteotomy. Foot Ankle Int 1999;20(3):167; with permission.) © 1996 by the American Orthopaedic Foot and Ankle Society.

Romash [62] described a calcaneal osteotomy through the plane of the primary fracture line with subtalar arthrodesis (Fig. 7). This restores calcaneal height and length, narrows the heel, and decompresses the lateral structures. It also addresses subtalar arthritis by arthrodesis.

The patient is placed in the lateral decubitus position. An oblique incision, in line with the skin creases, is made over the sinus tarsi. The approach is limited by the peroneal tendons and sural nerve inferiorly and branches of the superficial peroneal nerve and the long extensor tendons dorsally. The extensor digitorum brevis muscle is retracted distally, and fat in the sinus tarsi is excised. Retracting the peroneal tendons, the subtalar joint is opened and the soft tissues are stripped carefully of the lateral calcaneal wall in a subperiosteal fashion. A lamina spreader is placed in the sinus tarsi and the joint is distracted. The posterior articular surfaces of the talus and calcaneus are denuded, which allows identification of the primary fracture line. A Steinmann pin is placed into the calcaneus in the plane of the primary fracture line; its position is confirmed with intraoperative axial and lateral radiographs. Using the Steinmann pin as a guide, a straight osteotome is used to divide the primary fracture line. Ideally, the osteotomy exits the medial wall posterior and inferior to the neurovascular

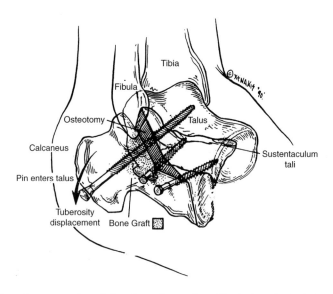

Fig. 7. Calcaneal osteotomy through the primary fracture line with subtalar arthrodesis for correction of severe deformity. (*From* Romash M. Reconstructive osteotomy of the calcaneus with subtalar arthrodesis for malunited calcaneal fractures. Clin Orthop 1993;290:165; with permission.)

structures. Extreme care should be taken to prevent injury to these structures, because the anatomy may be distorted. Temporary screw fixation of the talus to the sustentacular calcaneal fragment provides a more stable foundation for deformity correction. With the help of a lateral joint distractor (half pins in the lateral tibia and calcaneal tuberosity), as well as a lamina spreader in the osteotomy, the tuberosity fragment is now displaced posteriorly and medially along the plane of the osteotomy. This shift may require some time to allow the soft tissues to relax. If necessary, a Schanz pin can be placed percutaneously in the tuberosity fragment to help with manipulation. After adequate correction is verified with radiographs, two 4.0-mm or 4.5-mm partially threaded cannulated screws are used to secure the tuberosity fragment to the sustentacular fragment. Distraction is released, the temporary fixation screw is removed, and the subtalar joint surfaces are prepared for arthrodesis as described above. The joint is packed with bone graft. Subtalar arthrodesis is performed with a large fragment screw from the posteroinferior aspect of the calcaneal tuberosity, through the sustentacular fragment into the talus. Additional bone graft is packed around the arthrodesis site and the lateral gap that is created by the osteotomy, and the wound is closed in layers over a small suction drain.

For calcaneal malunions (Stephens type III) with a large lateral wall exostosis, subtalar arthritis, and more than 10° of axial hindfoot malalignment (varus more common than valgus), Sanders and colleagues recommended a lateral wall exostectomy, peroneal tenolysis, subtalar distraction bone block fusion, and a Dwyer-type calcaneal osteotomy [32,46]. The surgical technique is the same as described above for distraction bone block arthrodesis. In this scenario, however, a calcaneal osteotomy is performed before placement of the subtalar arthrodesis screws. A lateral closing wedge osteotomy is used to correct for severe varus deformities. In malunions with valgus deformity, a medializing calcaneal osteotomy with rotation of the tuberosity is recommended [46]. Simultaneous fixation of osteotomy and subtalar fusion is achieved with two partially threaded large fragment cannulated screws.

Summary

Calcaneus fracture malunions are disabling for the patient and challenging for the treating physician. Because of the multitude of problems that can occur, a careful clinical and radiographic evaluation is prudent. Similar to the treatment of acute calcaneal fractures, patient selection is critical and management has to be individualized. Realistic patient expectations and surgical goals must be discussed before any surgical intervention; despite the best efforts, restoration of a fully functional, pain-free foot rarely is possible. In most cases, function can be improved greatly by a carefully planned reconstructive surgical intervention.

References

[1] DiGiovanni C, Benirschke S, Hansen SJ. Foot injuries. In: Browner B, Jupiter J, Levine A, et al, editors. Skeletal trauma. 3rd edition. Philadelphia: WB Saunders Company; 2003. p. 2375–492.

[2] Hildebrand K, Buckley R, Mohtadi N, et al. Functional outcome measures after displaced intra-articular calcaneal fractures. J Bone Joint Surg 1996;78B(1):119–23.

[3] Cotton F. Old os calcis fractures. Ann Surg 1921;74:294–303.

[4] Bankart A. Fractures of the os calcis. Lancet 1942;2:175.

[5] Bohler L. Diagnosis, pathology, and treatment of fractures of the os calcis. J Bone Joint Surg 1931;13:75–89.

[6] Letournel E. Open reduction and internal fixation of calcaneal fractures. In: Spiegel P, editor. Topics in orthopaedic trauma. Baltimore (MD): University Park Press; 1984. p. 173–92.

[7] Benirschke SK, Sangeorzan BJ. Extensive intraarticular fractures of the foot. Clin Orthop 1993;292:128–34.

[8] Sanders R, Swiontkowski M, Nunley J, et al. The management of fractures with soft-tissue disruptions. Instr Course Lect 1994;43:559–70.

[9] Sanders R, Fortin P, Walling A. Subtalar arthrodesis following calcaneal fracture. Presented at the Annual Meeting of the American Association of Orthopaedic Surgeons. 1991.

[10] Buckley R, Tough S, McCormack R, et al. Operative compared with nonoperative treatment of displaced intra-articular calcaneal fractures: a prospective, randomized, controlled multicenter trial. J Bone Joint Surg 2002;84A(10):1733–44.

[11] Thermann H, Krettek C, Hufner T, et al. Management of calcaneal fractures in adults. Clin Orthop 1998;353:107–24.

[12] Essex-Lopresti P. The mechanism, reduction technique, and results in fractures of the os calcis. Br J Surg 1952;39(157):395–419.

[13] Sangeorzan B, Ananthakrishnan D, Tencer A. Contact characteristics of the subtalar joint after a simulated calcaneus fracture. J Orthop Trauma 1995;9(3):251–8.

[14] Tornetta III P. Percutaneous treatment of calcaneal fractures. Clin Orthop Relat Res 2000;(375):91–6.

[15] Zwipp H, Rammelt S. Posttraumatic deformity correction at the foot. Zentralbl Chir 2003; 128(3):218–26.

[16] Rammelt S, Zwipp H. Calcaneus fractures: facts, controversies and recent developments. Injury 2004;35(5):443–61.

[17] Rammelt S, Grass R, Zawadski T, et al. Foot function after subtalar distraction boneblock arthrodesis: a prospective study [lower limb]. J Bone Joint Surg 2004;86B(5):659–68.

[18] James E, Hunter G. The dilemma of painful old os calcis fractures. Clin Orthop 1983;177: 112–5.

[19] Sarrafian S. Anatomy of the foot and ankle. 2nd edition. Philadelphia: Lippincott Company; 1993.

[20] Rosenbaum D, Becker H-P. Plantar pressure distribution measurements. Technical background and clinical applications. Foot Ankle Surg 1997;3:1–14.

[21] Davies M, Betts R, Scott I. Optical plantar pressure analysis following internal fixation for displaced intra-articular os calcis fractures. Foot Ankle Int 2003;24(11):851–6.

[22] Hansen S. Posttraumatische Fehlstellung des RuckfuBes. Orthopade 1991;20:95–8.

[23] Macey L, Benirschke S, Sangeorzan B, et al. Acute calcaneal fractures: treatment options and results. J Am Acad Orthop Surg 1994;2(1):36–43.

[24] Isbister J. Calcaneo-fibular abutment following crush fracture of the calcaneus. J Bone Joint Surg Br 1974;56B(2):274–8.

[25] Mulcahy DM, Stephens MM. Intra-articular calcaneal fractures: effect of open reduction and internal fixation on contact characteristics of the subtalar joint. Foot Ankle 1998;19(12):842–8.

[26] Csizy M, Buckley R, Tough S, et al. Displaced intra-articular calcaneal fractures: variables predicting late subtalar fusion. J Orthop Trauma 2003;17(2):106–12.

[27] Borrelli JJ, Torzilli P, Grigiene R, et al. Effect of impact load on articular cartilage: development of an intra-articular fracture model. J Orthop Trauma 1997;11(5):319–26.

[28] Buch BD, Myerson MS, Miller SD. Primary subtalar arthrodesis for the treatment of comminuted calcaneal fractures. Foot Ankle Int 1996;17(2):61–70.

[29] Myerson M, Quill Jr G. Late complications of fractures of the calcaneus. J Bone Joint Surg 1993;75A(3):331–41.

[30] Paley D, Hall H. Intra-articular fractures of the calcaneus. A critical analysis of results and prognostic factors. J Bone Joint Surg 1993;75A(3):342–54.

[31] Pozo J, Kirwan E, Jackson A. The long-term results of conservative management of severely displaced fractures of the calcaneus. J Bone Joint Surg 1984;86B(3):386–90.

[32] Stephens H, Sanders R. Calcaneal malunions: results of prognostic computed tomography classification system. Foot Ankle Int 1996;17(7):395–401.

[33] Chandler J, Bonar S, Anderson R, et al. Results of in situ subtalar arthrodesis for late sequelae of calcaneus fractures. Foot Ankle Int 1999;20(1):18–24.

[34] Kamel R, Sakla F. Anatomical compartments of the sole of the human foot. Anat Rec 1961; 140:57–60.

[35] Manoli A, Weber T. Fasciotomy of the foot: an anatomical study with special reference to release of the calcaneal compartment. Foot Ankle 1990;10(5):267–75.

[36] Myerson M. Management of compartment syndromes of the foot. Clin Orthop 1991;271: 239–48.

[37] Jung H, Yoo M, Kim M. Late sequelae of secondary Haglund's deformity after malunion of tongue type calcaneal fracture: report of two cases. Foot Ankle Int 2002;23(11):1014–7.

[38] Anderson R, Pleimann J. Differentiating tibio-talar and subtalar joint pain prior to arthrodesis. Tech Foot Ankle Surg 2003;2(1):47–50.

[39] Finkbeiner G, Stohr C, Leemreijze P. Tarsaltunnelsyndrom und Trauma. Kasuisticher Beitrag zur Atiologie und Therapie. Monatsschar Unfallheilk 1975;78:269–74.

[40] Carr J, Hansen S, Benirschke S. Subtalar distraction bone block fusion for late complications of os calcis. Foot Ankle 1988;9(2):81–6.

[41] Bednarz P, Beals T, Manoli A. Subtalar distraction bone block fusion: an assessment of outcome. Foot Ankle Int 1997;18(12):785–91.

[42] Loucks C, Buckley R. Bohler's angle: correlation with outcome in displaced intra-articular calcaneal fractures. J Orthop Trauma 1999;13(8):554–8.

[43] Huang P, Fu Y, Cheng Y, et al. Subtalar arthrodesis for late sequelae of calcaneal fractures: fusion in situ versus fusion with sliding corrective osteotomy. Foot Ankle Int 1999;20(3):166–70.

[44] Flemister A, Infante A, Sanders R, et al. Subtalar arthrodesis for complications of intra-articular calcaneal fractures. Foot Ankle Int 2000;21(5):392–9.

[45] Ebraheim N, Zeiss J, Skie M, et al. Radiologic evaluation of peroneal tendon pathology associated with calcaneal fractures. J Orthop Trauma 1991;5(3):365–9.

[46] Clare M, Lee WR, Sanders R. Intermediate to long-term results of a treatment protocol for calcaneal fracture malunions. J Bone Joint Surg 2005;87A(5):963–73.

[47] Hansen S. Functional reconstruction of the foot and ankle. Philadelphia: Lippincott Williams & Wilkins; 2000.

[48] Robinson J, Murphy G. Arthrodesis as salvage for calcaneal malunions. Foot Ankle Clin 2002; 7:107–20.

[49] Braly W, Bishop J, Tullos H. Lateral decompression for malunited os calcis fracture. Foot Ankle 1985;6(2):90–6.

[50] Russotti G, Cass J, Johnson K. Isolated talocalcaneal arthrodesis. J Bone Joint Surg 1988; 70A(10):472–8.

[51] Mann R, Beamon D, Horton G. Isolated subtalar arthrodesis. Foot Ankle Int 1998;19(8):511–9.

[52] Dahm D, Kitakoa H. Subtalar arthrodesis with internal compression for post-traumatic arthritis. J Bone Joint Surg 1998;80B(1):134–8.

[53] Easley M, Trnka H-J, Schon L, et al. Isolated subtalar arthrodesis. J Bone Joint Surg 2000; 82A(5):613–24.

[54] Haskell A, Pfeiff C, Mann R. Subtalar joint arthrodesis using a single lag screw. Foot Ankle Int 2004;25(11):774–7.

[55] Hintermann B, Valderrabano V, Nigg B. Influence of screw type on obtained contact area and contact force in a cadaveric subtalar arthrodesis model. Foot Ankle Int 2002;23(11):986–91.

[56] Gallie W. Subastragalar arthrodesis in fractures of the os calcis. J Bone Joint Surg 1943; 25A:731–6.

[57] Amendola A, Lammens P. Subtalar arthrodesis using interposition iliac crest bone graft after calcaneal fracture. Foot Ankle Int 1996;17(10):608–14.

[58] Chan S, Alexander I. Subtalar arthrodesis with interposition tricortical iliac crest graft for late pain and deformity after calcaneus fracture. Foot Ankle Int 1997;18(10):613–5.

[59] Trnka H-J, Easley ME, Lam PW-C, et al. Subtalar distraction bone block arthrodesis. J Bone Joint Surg [Br] 2001;83B:849–54.

[60] Burton D, Olney B, Horton G. Late results of subtalar distraction fusion. Foot Ankle Int 1998; 19(4):197–202.

[61] Ishikawa S, Murphy G, Richardson E. The effect of cigarette smoking on hindfoot fusions. Foot Ankle Int 2002;23(11):996–8.

[62] Romash M. Reconstructive osteotomy of the calcaneus with subtalar arthrodesis for malunited calcaneal fractures. Clin Orthop 1993;290:157–67.

ELSEVIER
SAUNDERS

Foot Ankle Clin N Am
11 (2006) 105–119

FOOT AND
ANKLE CLINICS

Late Reconstruction After Navicular Fracture

Murray J. Penner, MD, BSc(MEng), FRCSC

*Division of Lower Extremity Reconstruction (Foot & Ankle), Department of Orthopaedics,
University of British Columbia, 590-1144 Burrard Street, Vancouver, British Columbia,
V6Z 2A5, Canada*

The tarsal navicular is the figurative and literal keystone of the medial longitudinal arch of the foot. Therefore, injuries to the navicular may have a disproportionately profound effect on the overall function of the foot and ankle in comparison with its small size. Even optimally treated injuries can go on to significant posttraumatic sequelae, and leave the midfoot with chronic deformity, arthritis, and loss of motion.

Fortunately, acute injuries to the midfoot in general, and the navicular specifically, are comparatively rare. At a major trauma center, over a period of 25 years, 50 navicular fractures were identified, for an average of only two per year [1]. Most of these rare injuries are of a complex nature, more than 70% are associated with subluxation or dislocation of Chopart's or Lisfranc's joints [1]. The rarity of these injuries results in a limited overall experience in their treatment. These factors, in conjunction with the typical complexity of these injuries, continue to make primary treatment challenging. Even with optimal treatment in the hands of experienced surgeons, outcomes often can be suboptimal [2].

When suboptimal outcomes occur after primary treatment, reconstructive procedures may be warranted in an effort to deal with the chronic posttraumatic sequelae of pain, deformity, and loss of function. The same factors that make primary treatment challenging (rarity, complex deformity, small bone size, easily compromised soft tissue envelope), contribute to making posttraumatic reconstruction equally or even more difficult.

Little has been written with respect to the posttraumatic reconstruction of navicular injuries [3,4]. Most often, information is presented as single case reports [5], or as a small part of a series dealing with talonavicular and midfoot

---

E-mail address: penner@burrardortho.com

reconstruction, in general [4]. This article reviews the posttraumatic sequelae that can be seen after navicular fracture and provides an overview of the treatment principles and alternatives that are available.

Navicular anatomy, biomechanics, and treatment principles

The tarsal navicular, also referred to as the tarsal scaphoid, takes its names from Latin and Greek terms, which mean "boat-shaped," respectively. This reflects its pyriform shape when viewed from posterior, the plantar-medial tuberosity (the bow), and the broader dorsal-lateral end (the stern). The proximal aspect is composed almost entirely of the cartilage-covered biconcave "socket" that articulates with the "dome" of the talar head. The distal surface of the navicular has three cartilage-covered articular facets, which are divided by two minor crests that articulate with the medial, middle, and lateral cuneiforms.

The joints that are formed by the navicular are of paramount importance to normal foot function. The talonavicular joint forms the major osseous component of the "acetabulum pedis" and its motion is coupled closely to the subtalar and calcaneocuboid joints [6]. The plantar calcaneonavicular ligament, or spring ligament, inserts onto the plantar aspect of the navicular to form the major static stabilizer of the talonavicular joint and the major ligamentous component of the "acetabulum pedis." Descriptions of the spring ligament have been variable [7]. The second major stabilizer is the lateral calcaneonavicular component of the bifurcate ligament, which extends from the anterior process of the calcaneus to the superior lateral aspect of the navicular. The combination of osseous and ligamentous structures allows for the rotational movement of the hindfoot around the talus as it is "cradled" within the acetabulum pedis. Disruption of any component of the acetabulum pedis may render the hindfoot unstable, whereas posttraumatic arthrosis or deformity may lead to significantly decreased motion and pain in the talonavicular joint. Loss of talonavicular motion through trauma or subsequent arthrodesis severely restricts overall hindfoot motion [8], and reduces subtalar motion by approximately 80% [6]. The effect of isolated talonavicular arthrodesis on hindfoot motion is much greater than that for isolated subtalar or calcaneocuboid arthrodesis, which leads to consideration of the talonavicular as an essential joint [9], second only to the ankle joint.

The naviculocuneiform joint has little motion; it is stabilized nearly rigidly by the strong plantar ligaments, which leads to its consideration as a nonessential joint [9]. Thus, at its distal aspect, the navicular serves as a stable base for the transverse tarsal arch and the longitudinal arch of the medial column of the foot. In addition, the bulk of the navicular serves as a "spacer," and maintains length of the medial column. In these respects, the navicular serves a critical, although mostly static, function.

These features lead to important treatment considerations. Reconstructive procedures should strive for preservation of the essential talonavicular joint wherever possible, in an effort to preserve hindfoot gait mechanics. Maintenance of the naviculocuneiform joint is not critical, whereas restoration of navicular length is paramount in maintaining the anatomic relationship between medial and lateral columns and subsequent midfoot alignment and function.

The navicular tuberosity is the major site of insertion of the posterior tibial tendon (PTT), the major dynamic stabilizer of the hindfoot and longitudinal arch [10]. An accessory navicular bone, which is present in 10% to 14% of feet, may lie at the posterior medial aspect of the tuberosity and assumes function as the main PTT insertion when present [11]. Trauma may lead to fracture of the navicular tuberosity or strain of the synchondrosis between the accessory navicular and the tuberosity, which may lead to potential loss of PTT function. Because this function is critical for normal foot mechanics, preservation or restoration of the navicular tuberosity and PTT insertion site is important in navicular reconstruction.

Vascularization of the navicular is from a large anastomotic network of branches from the dorsalis pedis and medial plantar arteries. These branches enter the bone circumferentially, but may leave the central portion of the navicular hypovascular [12]. High-energy trauma may strip large portions of soft tissue attachment away from the navicular, as can aggressive surgical dissection, which may compromise navicular blood supply. These factors should be considered in planning reconstructive approaches.

Navicular trauma variants

Navicular fractures can be divided into dorsal avulsion fractures, body fractures, and tuberosity fractures/accessory navicular synchondrosis strains. Dorsal avulsion fractures (Fig. 1) generally do not produce substantial posttraumatic sequelae that require reconstruction, although posttraumatic arthritis is possible.

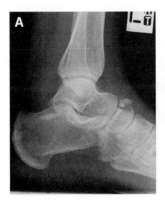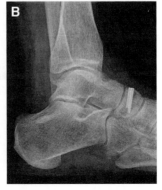

Fig. 1. Dorsal avulsion navicular fractures may involve a significant portion of the talonavicular joint surface (*A*), but anatomic fixation often is possible (*B*), which reduces the potential for major posttraumatic sequelae.

Navicular body fractures often result from higher energy mechanisms, such as axial loading or crushing of the midfoot. This can lead to substantial deformity of the navicular through fragment comminution and displacement, as well as substantial midfoot deformity. These fractures have been classified by Sangeorzan and colleagues [2] into three types with increasing severity and reduction difficulty. Type 1 fractures tend to be noncomminuted, with a transverse fracture line lying roughly in the plane of the metatarsals; this separates a dorsal fragment of the navicular from a larger plantar fragment. Often, primary treatment is able to restore the overall anatomy of the navicular well, and significant posttraumatic sequelae that require reconstruction are comparatively rare. As with any intra-articular fracture, posttraumatic arthritis may result, although major deformity is unusual.

Type 2 body fractures are the most common type, and result from axial compression with the forefoot being forced into dorsiflexion and adduction (Fig. 2). Typically, the fracture line runs from the dorsal lateral aspect of the navicular to the plantar medial aspect. A large dorsal medial fragment often is displaced medially, which allows subluxation of the talonavicular joint and shortening of the medial

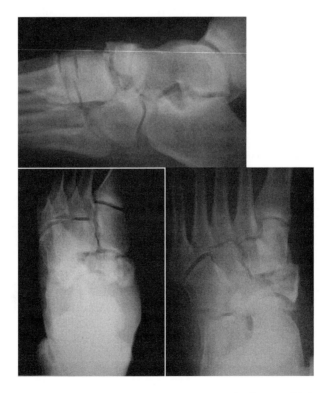

Fig. 2. Radiographs of an extensively comminuted type 2 navicular fracture with the typical large (but comminuted) dorsal medial fragment, dorsiflexion, mild adduction, and shortening of the medial column.

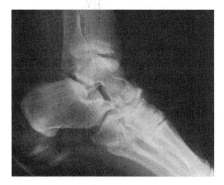

Fig. 3. Type 3 navicular burst fracture with severe comminution and medial column shortening. Typically, these are high-energy injuries that often are accompanied by injuries to the tarsometatar-sal, subtalar, and calcaneocuboid joints.

column. If associated with comminution, primary fracture treatment can be challenging, and may lead to late deformity and arthrosis that require reconstruction.

Type 3 body fractures are caused by axial compression with lateral deviation of the forefoot. This can be considered a burst fracture; the major fracture lines tend to lie in the middle and lateral portion of the navicular, generally with significant comminution and displacement (Fig. 3). An abduction deformity of the midfoot with medial column shortening may be seen, particularly when the medial navicular also is fragmented. If the medial navicular is grossly intact, the head of the talus may drop into the lateral navicular defect when the abducted forefoot is reduced. This may lead to a shortened medial column with forefoot adduction, as may be seen after type 2 fractures. Primary treatment of these fractures is difficult, with satisfactory results in less than 50% of cases [2]. Therefore, late reconstruction may be required.

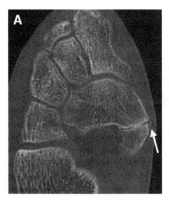
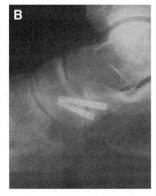

Fig. 4. A 28-year-old man who had an acute strain of an accessory navicular synchondrosis that was caused by a twisting crush injury. (A) Pain was localized to the medial aspect of the navicular tuberosity with associated focal uptake on bone scan and a subtle bony avulsion seen on CT scan (arrow). (B) The synchondrosis was debrided and fixed with two screws.

Tuberosity fractures and injuries to the accessory navicular synchondrosis usually are avulsion injuries that are caused by eversion of the foot with eccentric contraction of the PTT. Most are minimally displaced and can be treated nonoperatively with satisfactory results [13]. If an accessory navicular is present, such injuries may convert it from a previously asymptomatic state to a chronically symptomatic state [14]. Treatment of the chronically painful accessory navicular may involve simple excision. Recently, debridement of the synchondrosis with screw fixation and fusion of the accessory (Fig. 4) has been described [11]. If a tuberosity nonunion or accessory navicular remains symptomatic in association with pathologic pes planus, and nonoperative measures have failed, flatfoot reconstruction procedures may be required. Such procedures fall outside the scope of this article.

Clinical assessment

The goal of reconstruction after navicular trauma is to improve foot function, gait, and mobility through correction of deformity and painful arthrosis. Subsequently, the aim of clinical assessment is to localize arthrosis and to identify deformity, defining it as fixed, partially fixed, or flexible, if present. Examination should include assessment of stance and gait, with particular emphasis on identifying hindfoot alignment, medial arch configuration, and forefoot varus or valgus alignment relative to the hindfoot. Single-stance heel rise should be performed to assess dynamic hindfoot function. Nonweight-bearing examination should include identification of resting foot deformity, and the correctability of such deformity. Palpation is aimed at identifying areas of maximal tenderness to localize arthrosis. Range of motion of the ankle joint, subtalar joint, transverse tarsal joint, and forefoot should be evaluated.

Additionally, examination should identify other factors that may influence treatment outcome, and hence, choice of treatment. The presence of previous incisions, lacerations, skin grafts, or chronic soft tissue compromise—as may be associated with major crush injuries—should be noted. Sometimes, the soft tissue envelope may be so compromised as to preclude any reconstructive efforts. The presence of a gastrocnemius contracture should be noted. Motor function of the PTT, peroneal tendons, Achilles tendon, and anterior tibial tendon must be evaluated, because these are the major motors of the hindfoot. Assessment of sensation and vascular status is important, as for any foot examination.

Imaging

As with clinical assessment, the goal of imaging studies is to define posttraumatic deformity and arthrosis of the midfoot and the navicular. Standing anteroposterior (AP), lateral, and oblique views of both feet and standing AP, lateral, and mortise views of both ankles are required to allow for comparison and an estimate of the patient's preinjury alignment. Assessment of medial column length, navicular collapse, sag of the longitudinal arch, talonavicular subluxation, and forefoot adduction or abduction is important. The presence and location of any internal fixation devices should be noted.

A high-definition three-plane CT scan of the hindfoot and midfoot is required to assess navicular bone stock for the presence of collapse, nonunion, fragment size, or avascular necrosis (AVN). CT scan also is most able to identify early arthritic changes in joints of the hindfoot and midfoot. Occasionally, MRI scanning may be useful if AVN is a consideration and the viability of the navicular is in question.

Treatment of navicular fracture sequelae

Unsatisfactory outcomes after navicular fracture tend to be associated with types 2 and 3 fractures. Occasionally, fractures can be so highly comminuted and displaced that they may be considered acutely "nonreconstructable" [15], and suboptimal outcomes can be anticipated. Potential significant sequelae after navicular fracture include persistent midfoot pain and mid- and hindfoot stiffness, secondary to posttraumatic fibrosis. Crush injury also may be associated with primary nerve injury and compartment syndrome.

Bony complications include AVN, nonunion, posttraumatic arthritis, and malunion. Each of these can lead to significant foot deformity, primarily through medial column shortening.

Nonunion

Rates of nonunion following navicular fracture are not defined clearly, although nonunion is believed to be more common after fractures of increasing severity [2,15]. Fracture union may be partial or incomplete, and the degree to which the fracture is united may correlate with symptoms. Complete nonunion is likely to go on to late displacement of bone fragments and functional collapse of the navicular and medial column with late deformity. Nonunion may be more common in the central portion of the navicular where the vascular supply to bone is more tenuous.

In view of the limited literature to guide treatment of nonunion, general principles are used. For patients who have no deformity and have mild to moderate symptoms that are suggestive of the stable nonunion, nonoperative treatment with a stiff-soled rocker-forefoot shoe, with a custom orthotic to support the longitudinal arch, is recommended initially. Operative treatment is indicated for severe pain, despite appropriate nonoperative treatment, particularly when associated with significant posttraumatic arthritis or deformity (Fig. 5).

Operative treatment for nonunion of the navicular with minimal deformity and arthritis is aimed at achieving bony union. This situation is rare, because most nonunions are seen after high-grade fractures where deformity and arthritis are

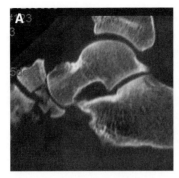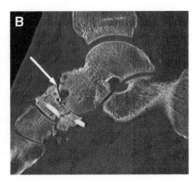

Fig. 5. Comminuted type 3 navicular fracture (*A*) that was fixed satisfactorily with restoration of medial column length (*B*). The patient had persistent mild to moderate pain 12 months postoperatively. CT scan shows partial undisplaced nonunion with degenerative changes in the talonavicular joint (*arrow*). The patient's symptoms were controlled reasonably with a stiff-soled rocker shoe and an orthotic. A talonavicular arthrodesis likely will be required at some point; because it is an essential joint, fusion will be deferred for as long as possible.

most likely. Nevertheless, if nonunion is found in the face of a functional talonavicular joint, revision open reduction with internal fixation with bone grafting is appropriate. Fusion of the fragments to the cuneiforms to increase fixation stability and bone mass of the fusion should be considered, because the naviculocuneiform joint is nonessential.

Before surgical treatment, low-grade infection must be ruled out as a potential cause of nonunion. Many of these injuries are associated with severe soft tissue compromise, and often, some degree of infection is present at some point in the course of treatment. Preoperative assessment with white blood cell count, erythrocyte sedimentation rate, and C-reactive protein is recommended on an empiric basis, and aspiration and culture of the nonunion site or talonavicular joint under fluoroscopic guidance may be useful. Intraoperative cultures should be obtained if a high degree of suspicion is present. In this situation, intravenous antibiotics should be maintained until cultures are negative at 5 days or for 6 weeks if the cultures prove to be positive.

The author's experience with treatment of isolated navicular nonunion with minimal deformity is limited and long-term outcomes have not been reported in the literature. Therefore, specific indications for treatment are lacking, and the decision to proceed to surgical treatment must be individualized. Treatment of nonunion with significant deformity is discussed below.

Avascular necrosis

AVN of the navicular may be partial or complete, and may occur despite optimal reduction and fixation. The limited blood supply to the central portion of the navicular has been implicated as a likely factor in the development of AVN; however, most navicular fractures are associated with major injuries to the soft tissues of the midfoot. Therefore, traumatic soft tissue stripping also seems likely to be a major contributor. Sangeorzan and colleagues [2] reported that 6 out of 21 fractures in their series developed AVN, and one went on to significant collapse. Some investigators have suggested that AVN may be most common after types 1 and 3 fractures [15], although no published series is large enough to gain a true sense of the overall incidence. Partial AVN may result in partial collapse of the lateral navicular preferentially [16]; this allows the talar head to drop into the lateral defect, and causes adduction through the talonavicular joint and shortening of the medial column. Therefore, the uninjured lateral column is long, and the hindfoot progresses into varus.

Diagnosis of AVN may be empiric, particularly if no collapse of the navicular is identified. Radiographs or CT scan images that demonstrate bony sclerosis may be indicative of early AVN, whereas frank collapse is strongly suggestive of AVN, particularly if this has been late in onset. MRI scan may be able to demonstrate AVN, but its usefulness typically is limited by the presence of internal fixation.

The literature does not offer clear guidance for the treatment of posttraumatic navicular AVN when collapse has not occurred. Idiopathic AVN of the navicular has been reported in adults (Fig. 6), but the controversy as to the nature of this entity is significant. For example, in the same journal volume, one report specifically distinguished AVN from Muller-Weiss syndrome, whereas the following

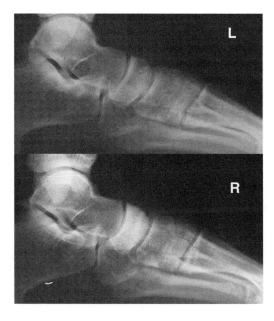

Fig. 6. Idiopathic AVN of the right navicular in a 30-year-old woman. She had no history of injury, only insidious onset of pain over the right navicular; bone scan and MRI scan findings support a diagnosis of AVN. Note the sclerosis of the right navicular (R) as compared with the left (L), with maintenance of medial column length and no collapse.

report specifically attributed Muller-Weiss syndrome to AVN [17,18]. As a result, treatment guidelines for posttraumatic AVN without collapse cannot be extrapolated from idiopathic AVN. With guidance from the literature lacking, treatment must be based on common principles. If AVN is present without collapse, but significant symptoms of pain are present and are attributable directly to the AVN, some effort to protect the navicular and offload it seems to be reasonable; however, because the duration that such intervention might be required is unknown, excessively restrictive measures do not seem to be warranted. Rather, optimized footwear, as noted for nonunions, together with recommendations against high impact, repetitive stress activities, seems to be the most reasonable.

If significant navicular collapse and foot deformity secondary to AVN occur, surgical intervention generally is required. This is discussed further below.

Posttraumatic arthritis

Posttraumatic talonavicular arthritis is the most common complication after navicular fracture [13]. A correlation between the quality of reduction of the articular surface of the navicular and posttraumatic arthritis has been described [2]. Arthritis may occur with gross collapse of the navicular, or occasionally, in the absence of marked navicular deformity (Fig. 6). Because most medial column motion occurs through the essential talonavicular joint, every effort should be made to preserve it for as long as possible, and nonoperative treatment should be maximized. At some point, nonoperative treatment may no longer suffice, and talonavicular arthrodesis with neutral alignment of the medial column and plantigrade positioning of the foot should be considered.

Because navicular injury often occurs in association with injuries to other joints of the midfoot, arthritis may not be confined to the talonavicular joint (Fig. 7). Extension of the arthrodesis to include the naviculocuneiform joints may be required. Preservation of the subtalar and calcaneocuboid joints, if they are not involved, seems to be most reasonable. Some motion in these joints, in principle, should be protective of the adjacent ankle joint; however, associated arthrosis in the subtalar or calcaneocuboid joints is not uncommon. Considering that talonavicular arthrodesis reduces motion in the subtalar joint by approximately 80% [6], exposing the patient to the risk of persistent hindfoot pain in an effort to preserve this last 20% of motion does not seem warranted in the presence of hindfoot arthrosis. In such cases, extension of the talonavicular arthrodesis to complete a triple arthrodesis is recommended (Fig. 8).

Isolated arthrodesis of the talonavicular joint (see Fig. 8) has been described by several investigators [19], and generally is regarded as technically demanding [20]. Although numerous technical variations are available, the general principles remain standard. Even when major navicular deformity is not present, maintenance of the length of the medial column of the foot must be considered. Resection of residual cartilage from the talonavicular joint, along with smoothing of posttraumatic irregularities in an effort to improve bony contact, may contribute to a few millimeters of shortening of the medial column. A high corre-

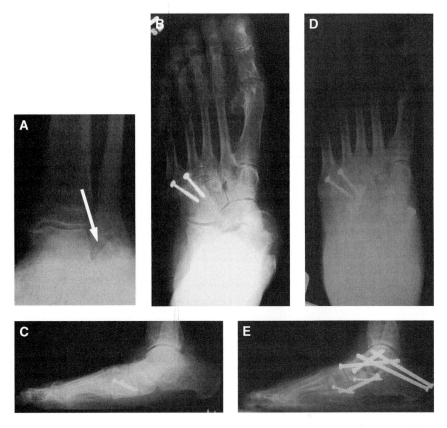

Fig. 7. Chronic subtalar (*A, arrow*) and talonavicular (*B, C*) fracture dislocation, 2 years after injury, with history of distant previous forefoot and midfoot surgeries. Extensive hindfoot traumatic arthrosis precluded isolated talonavicular arthrodesis; triple arthrodesis was performed successfully with realignment and restoration of medial column length (*D, E*).

lation between correct column length and good functional outcome has been shown in the treatment of midfoot injuries [1]. In addition to medial column length control, careful positioning of the talonavicular arthrodesis is critical, because most of the potentially compensatory motion of the hindfoot is lost with such fusions. Care must be taken to position the hindfoot in neutral to slight valgus and then position the mid- and forefoot in neutral alignment to the hindfoot. To prevent lateral border overload and pain, particular care must be taken to avoid forefoot varus.

The technique for talonavicular arthritis where bone loss is not significant begins with a medial approach between the anterior tibial tendon and the PTT. Thickened, fibrotic capsular tissue is anticipated in the posttraumatic setting when the talonavicular joint is exposed. Avoidance of excessive stripping of the soft tissues from the talar neck is recommended. Initially, the talonavicular joint is opened with a small elevator. Any remaining articular cartilage is scraped from

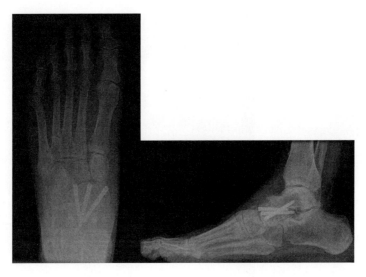

Fig. 8. Isolated talonavicular arthrodesis for posttraumatic arthritis. Note the minimal subtalar and calcaneocuboid arthrosis and maintenance of medial column length and alignment.

the subchondral bone using a small curved osteotome and angled curettes to get around the dome of the talar head. As dissection progresses, the joint relaxes, which allows insertion of a small lamina spreader and progressively better visualization of the lateral extent of the joint. This further serves to free up the joint, which facilitates reduction of the joint and alignment of the foot, before fixation. Care is taken to ensure that the subchondral bone is maintained, which guarantees minimal loss of medial column length. The subchondral surface is prepared for fusion with multiple perforations using a 1.6-mm drill or small burr.

The talonavicular joint is reduced and the foot is positioned with slight heel valgus and neutral forefoot rotation, which often requires active pronation of the forefoot to avoid positioning it in varus. Apposition of the talar head and navicular bone surfaces is assessed. If large defects preclude good bone–bone contact, a proximal tibial cancellous bone graft is inserted. The joint is stabilized provisionally with three 1.4-m guide wires. Position of the arthrodesis and guide wires is checked with fluoroscopy. Cannulated compression screws are used over the guide wires to ensure good interfragmentary compression and rigid stabilization. Depending on the size and quality of the bone, the specific size and type of fixation may need to be individualized. Further bone graft may be packed around the fusion site; this is followed by routine closure, wound dressing, and splinting. A cast or boot is used for 10 to 12 weeks, the first 6 weeks nonweight-bearing, and the last 6 weeks progressive weight-bearing as tolerated.

The results of talonavicular arthrodesis for posttraumatic arthritis of the talo-navicular joint have not been reported widely. In particular, the author found no specific reports that focused on arthrodesis after navicular fracture. Rather, a few cases are mentioned as complications in reports on acute navicular fracture [2], or are contained within reports of talonavicular arthrodesis, in general. The most applicable article is by Chen and colleagues [4], who reviewed 16 isolated talonavicular arthrodeses. Eight of these cases had posttraumatic arthritis, and three were noted specifically to be secondary to navicular fracture. Outcomes for these cases were not reported individually. As a group, 1 out of 16 cases went on to nonunion, and only 1 case was reported as unsatisfactory. They believed that isolated talonavicular arthrodesis was effective for the treatment of posttraumatic talonavicular arthritis.

Nonunion remains the most concerning complication after talonavicular arthrodesis. Although reported rates vary widely [20], nonunion typically is believed to occur in up to 10% of cases [19].

Medial column deformity

When significant navicular collapse is present secondary to nonunion, AVN, or simply a severe nonreconstructable fracture pattern, medial column shortening results (Fig. 9). Persistent foot pain and dysfunction may be anticipated, and generally are severe enough to warrant surgical reconstruction. Because preservation of the talonavicular joint is not possible in these situations, restoration of normal hindfoot mechanics is not possible; however, improvement in overall foot alignment with the specific aim of correcting column length discrepancies has been correlated with better functional outcomes [1].

Techniques for the restoration of medial column length using distraction talonavicular arthrodesis have been described by a few investigators [9,20]. The principles of talonavicular arthrodesis as outlined above are followed. Preoperative assessment of radiographs with comparison to the contralateral side is necessary to gain an estimate of the degree of bone loss and the likely size of bone graft that is required. Intraoperatively, the talonavicular joint is exposed and all nonviable bone is removed. The bone surfaces of the talar head proximally and any remaining navicular bone distally are cut parallel, which exposes viable cancellous bone. Using manual manipulation, a lamina spreader, or small pin distractor, the medial column is distracted out to its appropriate length. The position is checked to ensure a slight hindfoot valgus and a neutral forefoot, and overall bony alignment is visualized further with fluoroscopy. If deformity has been long-standing, the lateral column and subtalar joint may be stiff, which prevents adequate realignment. Formal release, realignment, and fusion of the subtalar and calcaneocuboid joints may be required. After satisfactory alignment has been achieved, the residual bony defect can be assessed, and a tricortical iliac crest bone block is harvested. It is pressed into position in the defect with a good friction fit between the prepared parallel surfaces. Typically, fixation of the fusion is performed with a medial small-fragment locking plate and interfragmentary screws where possible. As with any distraction arthrodesis, consolidation of the fusion mass is expected to be prolonged. The duration of cast immobilization, and weight-bearing status must be individualized based on radiographs and clinical assessment.

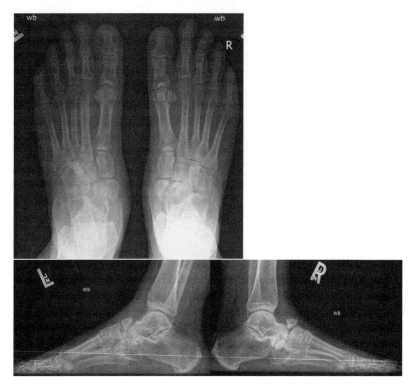

Fig. 9. Patient who had bilateral navicular fracture nonunions 14 months after external and K-wire fixation for bilateral grade 3 open Lisfranc, Chopart, and subtalar joint fracture dislocations that were sustained in a 30-foot fall. Although overall alignment is surprisingly good, note the loss of medial column length and resultant concave medial soft tissue shadows of both feet, which lead to a clinical appearance of forefoot adductus. Her symptoms were mild, and management has been non-operative. Operative management, when indicated, optimally would include distraction talonavicular arthrodesis to restore medial column length.

The author found no series which reported results specific to distraction talonavicular arthrodesis for navicular bone loss. Generally, such cases are noted as individual cases within a larger case series or chapter. As a result, a generalization of results cannot be provided; however, if fusion can be achieved and overall alignment of the foot can be restored through medial column lengthening, in principle, improvement in symptoms, shoe fitting, and function should be anticipated.

Summary

Although the need for late reconstruction after navicular fracture is not uncommon, the rarity of navicular fractures overall, and improving techniques in acute management mean that surgeon experience with late procedures typically is limited. Consequently, posttraumatic reconstruction of the navicular must be based on a sound understanding of principles, because no large body of published experience is available to guide treatment. The principles of restoring foot alignment and medial column length, together with good basic arthrodesis technique, are critical in obtaining satisfactory outcomes.

References

[1] Richter M, Wippermann B, Krettek C, et al. Fractures and fracture dislocations of the midfoot: occurrence, causes and long-term results. Foot Ankle Int 2001;22:392–8.

[2] Sangeorzan BJ, Benirschke SK, Mosca V, et al. Displaced intra-articular fractures of the tarsal navicular. J Bone Joint Surg 1989;71A:1504–10.

[3] Castro MD. Arthrodesis of the navicular. Foot Ankle Clin 2004;9:73–83.

[4] Chen CH, Huang PJ, Chen TB, et al. Isolated talonavicular arthrodesis for talonavicular arthritis. Foot Ankle Int 2001;22:633–6.

[5] Dhillon MS, Gupta R, Nagi ON. Inferomedial (subsustentacular) dislocation of the navicular: a case report. Foot Ankle Int 1999;20:196–200.

[6] Walker N, Stukenborg C, Savory KM, et al. Hindfoot motion after isolated and combined arthrodeses: measurements in anatomic specimens. Foot Ankle Int 2000;21:921–7.

[7] Golano P, Farinas O, Saenz I. The anatomy of the navicular and periarticular structures. Foot Ankle Clin 2004;9:1–23.

[8] Astion DJ, Deland JT, Otis JC, et al. Motion of the hindfoot after simulated arthrodesis. J Bone Joint Surg 1997;79A:241–6.

[9] Hansen Jr ST. Functional anatomy of the foot and ankle. In: Functional reconstruction of the foot and ankle. Philadelphia: Lippincott Williams & Wilkins; 2000. p. 17–32.

[10] Kitaoka HB, Luo ZP, An KA. Effect of the posterior tibial tendon on the arch of the foot during simulated weightbearing: biomechanical analysis. Foot Ankle Int 1997;18:43–6.

[11] Ugolini PA, Raikin SM. The accessory navicular. Foot Ankle Clin 2004;9:165–80.

[12] Torg J, Pavlov H, Cooley L, et al. Stress fractures of the tarsal navicular: a retrospective review of twenty-one cases. J Bone Joint Surg 1982;64A:700–12.

[13] Thordarson DB. Fractures of the midfoot and forefoot. In: Myerson MS, editor. Foot and ankle disorders. Philadelphia: WB Saunders; 2000. p. 1265–96.

[14] Coughlin MJ. Sesamoids and accessory bones of the foot. In: Coughlin MJ, Mann RA, editors. Surgery of the foot and ankle. 7th edition. St. Louis (MO): Mosby; 1999. p. 437–99.

[15] DiGiovanni CW. Fracture of the navicular. Foot Ankle Clin 2004;9:25–63.

[16] Sanders R. Fractures of the midfoot and forefoot. In: Coughlin MJ, Mann RA, editors. Surgery of the foot and ankle. 7th edition. St. Louis (MO): Mosby; 1999. p. 1574–605.

[17] Maceira E, Rochera R. Muller-Weiss disease: clinical and biomechanical features. Foot Ankle Clin 2004;9:105–25.

[18] Sizensky JA, Marks RM. Imaging of the navicular. Foot Ankle Clin 2004;9:181–209.

[19] Sammarco GJ, Chang L. Talonavicular arthrodesis. In: Kitaoka HB, editor. Master techniques in orthopedic surgery: the foot and ankle. 2nd edition. Philadelphia: Lippincott Williams & Wilkins; 2002. p. 253–63.

[20] Castro MD. Arthrodesis of the navicular. Foot Ankle Clin 2004;9:73–83.

ELSEVIER
SAUNDERS

Foot Ankle Clin N Am
11 (2006) 121–126

FOOT AND
ANKLE CLINICS

Management of Cuboid Crush Injuries

Robert M. Mihalich, MD[a],*, John S. Early, MD[b,c]

[a]Department of Orthopedics, Baylor University Medical Center,
411 North Washington Avenue, Suite 7000, Dallas, TX 75246, USA
[b]Texas Orthopaedic Associates LLP, 8210 Walnut Hill Lane, Suite 130, Dallas, TX 75231, USA
[c]Orthopaedic Surgery, University of Texas Southwestern Medical Center, 8210 Walnut Hill Lane,
Suite 130, Dallas, TX 75231, USA

Injuries to the lateral column of the foot can involve the anterior aspect of the calcaneus, the cuboid, and the fourth and fifth metatarsals. These injuries are often associated with injuries of the medial column as well, many of which demonstrate operative indications. Isolated injuries of the lateral column, more specifically, the cuboid, are rare but have been described. Missed fractures or nonoperative treatment of displaced cuboid injuries can lead to shortening of the lateral column with subsequent flatfoot deformity, which may be painful. This article summarizes the scope of the problem and describes current treatment recommendations.

Mechanism of injury

Several mechanisms of injury and fracture patterns have been described. The classic "nutcracker" fracture described by Hermel and Gershon-Cohen [1] results from forced plantar flexion and abduction crushing the cuboid between the calcaneus and fourth and fifth metatarsals. The crushed cuboid shortens the lateral column and can include fractures extending into the proximal and distal articular surfaces. The short lateral column changes the weight-bearing position of the foot under the talus. Intra-articular step-off results in incongruent joints and possibly early arthrosis, especially in the mobile fourth and fifth tarsometatarsal joints.

---

* Corresponding author.
E-mail address: rmihalich@charter.net (R.M. Mihalich).

Alternatively, plantar flexion and abduction of the forefoot can impact the dorsolateral aspect of the articular facets of the fourth and fifth metatarsals into the cuboid. This injury may not necessarily result in shortening of the lateral column but can cause arthrosis. Weber and Locher [2] reported the largest series of cuboid fractures and observed this pattern in 11 of 12 patients. Five of the 12 patients had an additional crush component that resulted in shortening of the lateral column.

A distraction force across the lateral aspect of the midfoot can result in avulsion type fractures that tend to be more common but result in fewer long-term problems than the compressive type injury of the cuboid.

Sequelae of lateral column injury

Malunion of a cuboid fracture can cause poor outcomes. Shortening of the lateral column can result in a flatfoot deformity. This defect may be symptomatic and have all of the attributes of the more commonly seen flatfoot associated with posterior tibial tendon insufficiency.

Disruption of the articular surfaces around the cuboid can result in painful arthrosis, deformity, and stiffness. The cuboid articulates with the calcaneus, fourth and fifth metatarsals, lateral cuneiform, and navicular. In the few reports describing this injury, articular involvement was seen in all compression type fractures of the cuboid [2,3]. The tarsometatarsal joints are especially problematic because they provide the majority of dorsiflexion/plantar flexion motion in the lateral column. This motion acts as a shock absorber to dissipate the normal forces generated with weight bearing.

Treatment

Nondisplaced fractures around the cuboid can be treated nonoperatively with immobilization, with or without restriction of weight bearing. Nevertheless, further imaging may be required to determine that the fracture is truly non-displaced. With plain films, the lateral column is best visualized with a medial oblique radiograph of the foot. In addition, a fracture or dislocation of the medial column should be ruled out. Failure to recognize instability or injury in the medial column can lead to significant long-term problems with lateral column stability. A CT scan is often indicated to image the entire midfoot, even in injuries that initially appear minimally or nondisplaced (Fig. 1).

In cases of lateral column shortening or articular displacement, operative reconstruction is advised. Surgical treatment should restore the lateral column length and plantar support of the midfoot. Surrounding joints must be restored to maintain the articular congruity and mobility at the fourth and fifth tarsometatarsal joints and calcaneocuboid joint.

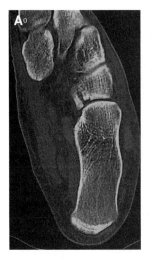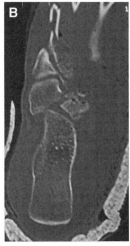

Fig. 1. (*A*) CT scan of a stable cuboid fracture not requiring operative intervention. (*B*) CT scan showing an impaction injury of the cuboid with loss of position. This injury requires operative intervention.

A lateral longitudinal incision is made proximal to the sural nerve from the angle of Gissane to just beyond the interval between the fourth and fifth metatarsals [4]. This incision allows access to the calcaneocuboid and tarsometatarsal joints. The cuboid position relative to the lateral cuneiform can be assessed. Dissection is carried down to bone. Subperiosteal dissection of the soft tissues exposes the articular surfaces and the lateral wall of the cuboid. An external fixator or distractor is required to restore the length of the lateral column. Fixation pins are placed in the anterior process of the calcaneus and in the fourth and fifth metatarsal shafts. The base of the metatarsals must line up appropriately when applying the fixator, because in-line distraction will reduce the cuboid articular surface. Initially, the lateral column is overdistracted to allow access to the articular surfaces for inspection and reduction [2,5] (Fig. 2).

Usually, only one articular surface of the cuboid is impacted or comminuted, equally affecting the calcaneocuboid joint or the tarsometatarsal joint surfaces. Starting from the medial fragments, the affected articular surface should be reconstructed using the intact side of the joint as a model. Once the articular surfaces are reassembled, the distraction device can be detensioned to the desired lateral column length. The large central void is filled with bone graft to help stabilize the articular ends and provide adequate scaffolding for compressive strength. Cancellous graft alone is used if the lateral wall is sufficiently intact and able to provide structural integrity to the cuboid once it is reduced into place. In injuries with increased lateral wall comminution, structural corticocancellous graft is needed to maintain proper cuboid length. Sangeorzan and Swiontkowski [3] described the use of corticocancellous iliac crest graft to reconstruct the lateral wall of the cuboid in two of four cases in their series. In one case, a three-hole

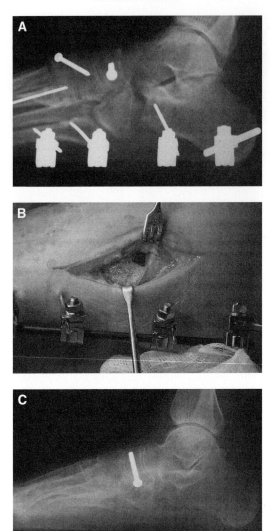

Fig. 2. (*A*) Preoperative view of impacted cuboid with external fixator in place for which re-construction was delayed owing to soft tissue injury medially. (*B*) Intraoperative view of fracture from lateral incision. (*C*) Two-year postoperative weight-bearing lateral view. No fixation was used in the cuboid. Reduction was supported by 6 weeks with a fixator in place on the lateral side.

one-third tubular plate was used as a buttress. Weber and Locher required iliac crest blocks of bone for 7 of 12 of the fractures in their series [2].

Fixation for this fracture depends on the degree of comminution. If the lateral wall can hold screws, 2.7 or 2.0 mm screws with or without minifragment plates can be used to secure the fracture reduction. Sanders recommends that the lateral column be held out to length with the use of a cervical H-plate [5], whereas Weber and Locher use two 2.0 mm plates placed dorsolaterally and plantar laterally to stabilize the construct [2]. In an injured foot with inadequate local bone integrity, a spanning internal fixator can be used in the form of a small fragment plate between the anterior aspect of the calcaneus and the lateral metatarsals. This fixator will hold the reduction and prevent any collapse during healing owing to peroneal brevis contracture. Implants used in this manner should normally be removed in 6 months but only after the patient has returned to weight bearing [5]. When soft tissue injury or extensive comminution tempers the desire to use an internal plate, the external fixator used for closed or limited open reduction can be left in place to hold length while the bone heals. The fixator is usually removed at 8 to 10 weeks and before any weight bearing. Postoperative treatment is similar to the nonoperative protocol, with initial immobilization for 6 weeks and non–weight bearing 10 to 12 weeks.

There are no published indications for immediate fusion of the calcaneocuboid or tarsometatarsal joints in the treatment of this injury. Late reconstruction of a cuboid crush injury and the resultant planovalgus deformity follows the same treatment principles. Reconstruction of the lateral column follows the same goals and outline as acute management. Initially, the lateral column length is restored and the fourth and fifth tarsometatarsal joints reconstructed. An external fixator is used to distract the cuboid until anatomy is restored. Occasionally, a contracted peroneus brevis tendon may prevent reduction. A lengthening of the brevis tendon at its musculotendinous junction posterior to the fibula just proximal to the syndesmosis may be required.

Once healed, reconstruction of a crushed cuboid and a short lateral column will require a distraction and arthrodesis of the calcaneocuboid joint. Although not ideal, loss of motion at the calcaneocuboid joint does not greatly affect the overall motion of the subtalar complex [6]. Fusion of the lateral tarsometatarsal joints should be avoided if possible. Despite literature supporting successful pain reduction with fusion of these joints, that opinion seems to be in the minority [7]. Interposition arthroplasty with silicon balls or rolled allograft or tendon autograft would allow continued motion and is preferable to fusion [8].

Concomitant medial column injuries may need late reconstruction. Careful assessment of the medial column is important when assessing the late sequelae of cuboid impaction injuries. Instability or valgus deviation at the medial tarso-metatarsal joints may be present and should be addressed during reconstruction to restore normal forefoot alignment. Realignment and fusion of the medial tarsometatarsal joints or navicular cuneiform joints will achieve these goals.

Summary

The major impact of a cuboid crush injury is the loss of structural integrity of the lateral column of the foot and the loss of motion at the lateral tarsometatarsal joints. Treating this injury, whether recognized early or late, usually requires operative intervention to preserve foot stability and function.

References

[1] Hermel MB, Gershon-Cohen J. Nutcracker fracture of the cuboid by indirect violence. Radiology 1953;60:850–4.
[2] Weber M, Locher S. Reconstruction of the cuboid in compression fractures: short to midterm results in 12 patients. Foot Ankle Int 2002;23(11):1008–13.
[3] Sangeorzan BJ, Swinontkowski MF. Displaced fractures of the cuboid. J Bone Joint Surg 1990; 72-B:376–8.
[4] Early JS. Fractures and dislocations of the midfoot and forefoot. Philadelphia: Lippincott, Williams and Wilkins; 2001.
[5] Sanders R. Fractures of the midfoot and forefoot. St. Louis: Mosby; 1999.
[6] Sands A, Early JS, Harrington RM, et al. Effect of variations in calcaneocuboid fusion technique on kinematics of the normal hindfoot. Foot Ankle Int 1998;19(1):19–25.
[7] Raikin SM, Schon LC. Arthrodesis of the fourth and fifth tarsometatarsal joints of the midfoot. Foot Ankle Int 2004;24(8):584–9.
[8] Berlet G, Anderson R. Tendon arthroplasty for basal fourth and fifth metatarsal arthritis. Foot Ankle Int 2002;23(5):440–4.

Foot Ankle Clin N Am
11 (2006) 127–142

FOOT AND
ANKLE CLINICS

Treatment of the Missed Lisfranc Injury

Michael S. Aronow, MD

*Department of Orthopaedic Surgery, University of Connecticut Health Center, Medical Arts and
Research Building, 263 Farmington Avenue, Farmington, CT 06034-4037, USA*

Ligament injuries and fractures that involve the tarsometatarsal (TMT), or Lisfranc, joints may lead to chronic pain and functional loss due to arthritis, deformity, or residual ligamentous instability, and associated soft tissue injury. It is well accepted that "significantly" displaced or unstable Lisfranc injuries are treated ideally with anatomic realignment and stabilization of the Lisfranc joints by way of open or closed techniques to decrease the incidence of these sequelae. Because of the lack of awareness about this injury, inadequate diagnostic evaluation, or patients not seeking medical care, the diagnosis of a Lisfranc injury may be "missed." This article discusses the management of these injuries when they are no longer acute.

Anatomy and biomechanics

The TMT joints consist of the five metatarsals and their articulation with the corresponding cuneiforms and cuboid. TMT joint stability comes from a combination of bone morphology, ligaments, and soft tissue support. The second metatarsal base forms a keystone with all three cuneiforms. The metatarsal bases, cuneiforms, and cuboid are wedge-shaped bones that form a stable "Roman arch" configuration. Ligaments cross the TMT, naviculocuneiform, and inter-cuneiform joints. Ligaments connect the second through fifth metatarsal bases, but not the first and second. The strong interosseous Lisfranc ligament connects the medial cuneiform to the medial second metatarsal base. There is a plantar ligament from the medial cuneiform to the plantar aspect of the second and third metatarsal bases and a weaker dorsal ligament from the medial cuneiform to the medial second metatarsal base [1,2]. Additional plantar arch support comes from

---

E-mail address: aronow@nso.uchc.edu

the intrinsic foot muscles; the plantar fascia; and the posterior tibial, anterior tibial, and peroneus longus tendons.

The first, second, and third TMT joints undergo slight dorsiflexion, plantarflexion, supination, and pronation motion that helps to absorb shock. They principally function as a rigid lever that connects the hindfoot to the forefoot. The fourth and fifth TMT joints have more motion which accommodate the forefoot on uneven terrain [3].

In a Lisfranc injury, there is instability, subluxation, or dislocation of the TMT joints secondary to ligament disruption and/or bone fracture. There may be ligamentous instability of the intercuneiform and naviculocuneiform joints. Associated fractures include the nutcracker impaction fracture of the cuboid, avulsion fracture of the navicular tuberosity, and fractures of the metatarsal bases. In most displaced Lisfranc injuries the weak dorsal TMT ligaments are disrupted first. The stronger plantar and interosseous ligaments rupture later, which in conjunction with more substantial plantar soft tissue support, causes dorsal displacement of the metatarsals. All five metatarsals may sublux laterally or medially in the transverse plane. Alternatively, the first metatarsal may sublux medially and/or some or all of the lateral four metatarsals may sublux laterally.

Mechanism of injury

Lisfranc injuries occur by direct and indirect mechanisms. Motor vehicle accidents and crush injuries are examples of dorsally or plantarly directed blows with a rotational component. The indirect mechanism of injury involves an axial force to a plantarflexed foot, usually with subsequent external rotation of the forefoot. Clinical examples include a fall on the stairs, a player landing on the posterior heel of an athlete's plantarflexed foot, and abduction of a foot fixed in a stirrup in equestrian and windsurfing injuries.

Clinical evaluation of acute Lisfranc injuries

In severe injuries with dislocation of the TMT joints there usually is significant pain, swelling, deformity, inability to bear weight, possible neurovascular compromise, and obvious radiographic findings. These injuries are rarely missed, with the possible exception of the patient who has experienced polytrauma, in whom a proper foot evaluation may be overlooked.

In subtle injuries there is pain, swelling, and tenderness, which often is limited to the area over the Lisfranc ligament. Weight-bearing is painful, but often possible. There may be a plantar ecchymosis sign [4] or a gap sign [5], a diastasis between the hallux and second toe. There may be no deformity or loss of the medial longitudinal arch with weight bearing only. TMT joint malalignment or instability may not be present or noticed on nonweight-bearing foot radiographs. Standard anteroposterior (AP) foot radiographs do not show the TMT joints clearly because they are taken perpendicular to the sole of the foot and not parallel to the TMT joint surfaces. The patient may present at a walk-in clinic, emergency room, or primary care provider's office where subtle physical examination and radiological findings may be missed. Orthopedic surgeons and podiatrists who are familiar with the disorder also may misdiagnose a Lisfranc injury if appropriate radiographic studies that demonstrate the ligamentous instability were not performed. The author has seen a case in which an acute asymmetric flat foot deformity secondary to a Lisfranc injury was misdiagnosed as posterior tibial tendon dysfunction because no foot radiographs were obtained, only an MRI of the ankle.

Clinical presentation of missed Lisfranc injuries

Missed Lisfranc injuries may present weeks to years after the injury has occurred, but before posttraumatic arthritis has set in. The patient may have delayed or foregone medical treatment for what was considered to be a routine "foot sprain." Alternatively, there may have been a delay in obtaining or interpreting appropriate diagnostic imaging studies correctly after acute evaluation with the diagnosis often not made by the original treating physician.

The patient also may present with a remote history of a foot injury and midfoot arthritis or deformity. The initial foot injury usually was considered minor, such as tripping over a coffee table. The patient may not have sought medical attention or was misdiagnosed as having a sprain. There may be progressive discomfort and deformity from the time of injury or a delay of several years before symptom development. The arthritis and deformity may be secondary to chondrocyte injury at the time of injury, residual joint incongruity, and ligamentous instability. The differential diagnosis includes idiopathic osteoarthritis, inflammatory arthritis, and neuropathic Charcot arthropathy.

The symptoms of patients who have subacute missed Lisfranc injuries depend upon the extent of the initial injury, how long ago it occurred, and the amount of interval ligamentous healing. There may be pain with, and limitations of, athletic activity or reduced walking tolerance. There may be deformity that ranges from a residual gap sign to an asymmetric flatfoot deformity with increased dorsiflexion and abduction at the TMT joints weight bearing. There may be inability to maintain arch during a single-leg heel raise. There may be tenderness over the TMT joints, particularly the second, and over the Lisfranc ligament. Midfoot abduction or adduction stress or divergent stress of the first and second metatarsals may cause pain.

Generally, the symptoms of patients who have more chronic missed Lisfranc injuries are related to the extent of midfoot deformity and arthritis. Tenderness and bossing may exist over the TMT, naviculocuneiform, or calcaneocuboid joints. An asymmetric midfoot-based flatfoot deformity—or less commonly, a midfoot adduction and plantarflexion deformity—may be present. There may be an antalgic gait with decreased push-off strength.

Imaging

Weight-bearing AP, lateral, and 30° oblique radiographs should be taken with the x-ray beam angled parallel to the TMT joint surfaces for the AP and 30° oblique views, the ankle in dorsiflexion, and the knee in extension. This angle gives a clearer view of the TMT joints, averages about 17° from perpendicular to the floor, and can be determined for any given individual on their lateral radiograph. TMT joint subluxation that is associated with chronic Lisfranc joint instability may be absent on radiographs that are taken nonweight-bearing, and sometimes even on radiographs that are taken full weight-bearing without dorsiflexion stress on the midfoot secondary to tensioning of a tight gastrocnemius/soleus complex. The author has observed that in some cadaver specimens with complete transection of the TMT and Lisfranc ligaments, TMT subluxation occurs with weight-bearing stress only with simulated triceps surae load and ankle dorsiflexion.

If weight-bearing radiographs do not show subluxation or dislocation, then stress radiographs should be taken to rule out ligamentous instability. Stress radiographs are obtained by stabilizing the cuboid and medial cuneiform and performing AP views while abducting and subsequently adducting all five metatarsals, and then displacing the first and second metatarsals divergently. Stress radiographs are more accurate if performed under anesthesia or an ankle block.

MRI and CT may show subtle fractures or joint incongruity that is not seen by plain radiograph [6,7]. The amount of TMT joint subluxation may be underestimated if the study is performed without simulated weight-bearing. MRI may show Lisfranc ligament injury or disruption and associated posterior tibial tendon or spring ligament pathology. CT scan can assess the extent of midfoot arthritis and bone loss. Depending upon the time since injury, bone scans may demonstrate posttraumatic arthritis or persistent instability that is related to Lisfranc ligament insufficiency.

Criteria for Lisfranc instability/malalignment

With rare exception [8], most studies suggest that outcome after Lisfranc injury improves with the quality of TMT joint reduction [9–25]. Multiple radiographic criteria for defining "unacceptable" displacement of an acute Lisfranc joint injury have been proposed; however, the amount of radiographic subluxation or displacement that exceeds the normal range or is associated with a poorer functional outcome has not been definitively determined.

The indications for surgical intervention in acute Lisfranc injuries and the accuracy of reduction have been based, in part, on the distance between the first and second metatarsal bases [12,14,16,19,20,22–24,26–29]. The criterion for an anatomic reduction ranged from a first–second metatarsal distance of less than or equal to 2 mm [12,20,22,23,26] to up to 5 mm [16,24]. Two of these studies measured the first–second metatarsal distance in the foot with a Lisfranc injury and the presumably normal contralateral foot. The distance in the injured feet ranged from 2 to 5 mm, whereas the distance in the uninjured feet averaged 1.3 mm [26] or ranged from 1 mm to 5 mm [27].

Although the distance between the lateral border of the medial cuneiform and the medial border of the second metatarsal reflects more directly the disruption of the Lisfranc ligament anatomically, it is used less often. In one study in which MRI and weight-bearing radiographs were taken of the injured and normal foot, the normal medial cuneiform–second metatarsal distance ranged from 2 mm to 5 mm. In 18 patients who had MRI-determined partial Lisfranc ligament tears it ranged from 1 mm less to 3 mm more than on the normal side. In 3 patients who had complete Lisfranc ligament ruptures, it was at least 2 mm greater than in the uninjured foot [27].

Malalignment of the first and second TMT joints may be visualized on the AP radiograph and at the third and fourth TMT joints on the 30° oblique view [30]. The medial and lateral aspects of the medial three metatarsal should line up with the corresponding cuneiforms. The medial aspect of the fourth metatarsal should line up with the medial aspect of the cuboid. In most Lisfranc injuries, at least one of the medial two TMT joints shows malalignment. The exception is isolated injuries to the medial–intermediate intercuneiform and Lisfranc ligaments in which only the medial cuneiform–second metatarsal and first–second metatarsal distances are increased. Open reduction and internal fixation (ORIF) has been recommended for 2 mm or more of displacement of any of the TMT joints [31]. In cadavers, 1 mm of dorsolateral displacement of the second metatarsal relative to the intermediate cuneiform produced an average of 13.1% decreased TMT joint contact, 2 mm of dorsolateral displacement produced an average of 25.5% decreased joint contact, and 4 mm of dorsolateral displacement produced an average of 50.6% decreased joint contact [32].

On an AP abduction stress radiograph, Lisfranc's ligament disruption is likely if a line drawn tangential to the medial aspect of the medial cuneiform and navicular does not intersect the first metatarsal base [33].

On the lateral radiograph the dorsal and plantar aspects of the metatarsals should line up with the corresponding cuneiform or cuboid. Faciszewski and colleagues [26] believed that patients who had Lisfranc injuries and flattening of the longitudinal arch had a poor prognosis and should undergo ORIF. Their criteria were the plantar aspect of the medial cuneiform being plantar to the plantar fifth metatarsal base or the medial cuneiform–fifth metatarsal base distance being 1.5 mm greater than in the contralateral foot. Myerson and colleagues [20] recommended open reduction if the lateral talo–first metatarsal angle was greater than 15°; however, these lateral radiograph findings may be seen in patients who have asymptomatic, atraumatic flatfoot deformities.

The author considers a medial cuneiform–second metatarsal distance of 2 mm or greater than on the normal contralateral side, or TMT subluxation of 2 mm or more, as an indication for surgical intervention in acute and symptomatic "missed" Lisfranc injuries.

Treatment options

Treatment options for the missed Lisfranc injury include nonoperative treatment, TMT joint realignment with joint preservation, arthrodesis, and arthroplasty. The goal is to obtain a minimally painful functional foot. Theoretically, this requires anatomic alignment of the midfoot joints and restoration of normal ligamentous stability. This preserves mechanical integrity of the arch and allows physiologic motion to dissipate load through the minimally mobile first, second, and third TMT joints [34]. Some patients are functional and asymptomatic despite residual foot deformity or arthritis. Alternatively, concurrent soft tissue injury, articular cartilage loss, and chondrocyte damage may result in persistent pain and arthritis despite anatomic TMT joint realignment.

Surgical TMT joint realignment may be associated with inadequate reduction, recurrent ligamentous instability after hardware removal, further articular cartilage damage from intra-articular screws or k-wires, and prominent hardware. There may be complications, including nerve injury, wound problems, and infection.

Joint arthrodesis offers relief of arthritic pain and avoidance of recurrent joint instability at the expense of joint motion, which may be a small price to pay for the medial three TMT and intercuneiform joints; however, fusion may be associated with a longer recovery time, nonunion, malunion with possible transfer metatarsalgia, and arthritis or deformity at adjacent joints. There also are the same issues that are seen with joint realignment procedures (eg, painful hardware, nerve damage, infection, wound problems).

Nonoperative treatment

Immobilization in a cast or cam walker may be particularly helpful to promote ligament healing in patients whose injuries are only a few weeks or months old. An insole orthosis or University of California Biomechanical Laboratory brace can support the arch, accommodate fixed deformity, limit subluxation that is due to ligamentous instability, and decrease painful motion of arthritic joints. A shoe with a stiff rocker sole or cane may aid ambulation. Acetaminophen, glucosamine/chondroitin sulfate, and nonsteroidal anti-inflammatory medication may be taken for pain or arthritis. Arthritic joints may note transient benefit from corticosteroid or hyaluronic acid injections. The patient may limit or avoid aggravating activities.

Joint realignment procedures

Joint reconstruction is a viable option for patients who have residual Lisfranc joint instability or subluxation and minimal to mild arthritis (Fig. 1). The surgical principles are the same as for acute Lisfranc injuries, with the possible exception of a decreased role for closed reduction and internal fixation. It may still be possible to percutaneously reduce and stabilize the second metatarsal to the medial cuneiform. However, if the Lisfranc ligament has already healed in an elongated fashion or if interposed scar tissue is being forcibly compressed by the screw, there will likely be recurrent subluxation and instability after hardware removal or failure.

Open reduction is performed through one or two dorsal longitudinal incisions. Depending on the extent of pathology, the first incision is made over the second TMT joint or between the first and second TMT joints. The first TMT joint may be exposed medial to the extensor hallucis longus tendon, avoiding injury to the dorsal medial cutaneous branch of the superficial peroneal nerve. Alternatively, the first TMT joint may be exposed in the interval between the

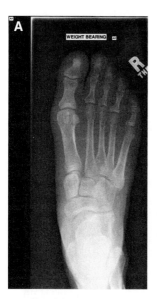
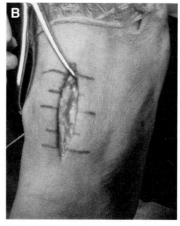

Fig. 1. 69-year-old man who sustained a right Lisfranc injury in a motor vehicle accident. The diagnosis was missed when he was evaluated at a local emergency room. ORIF was performed 2 months after injury. (*A*) AP foot radiograph showing an increased medial cuneiform–second metatarsal distance and subluxation of the medial border of the second metatarsal base relative to the medial aspect of the intermediate cuneiform. (*B*) Intraoperative reduction using a clamp between the medial cuneiform and the second metatarsal. A cannulated screw guide wire was placed across the area where the Lisfranc ligament connects the medial cuneiform and the second metatarsal avoiding the articular cartilage of the first TMT and medial–intermediate intercuneiform joints. (*C*) Anatomic alignment of the second and third TMT joints has been obtained as visualized in the interval between the extensor hallucis brevis and extensor digitorum longus tendon to the second toe. (*D*) Postoperative AP foot radiograph showing reduction of the medial cuneiform–second metatarsal distance and alignment of the medial border of the second metatarsal base relative to the medial aspect of the intermediate cuneiform. (*E*) Postoperative 30°-oblique foot radiograph showing alignment of the third TMT joint and the medial border of the fourth metatarsal base relative to the medial aspect of the cuboid. (*F*) Postoperative lateral foot radiograph showing alignment of the dorsal borders of the first and second TMT joints.

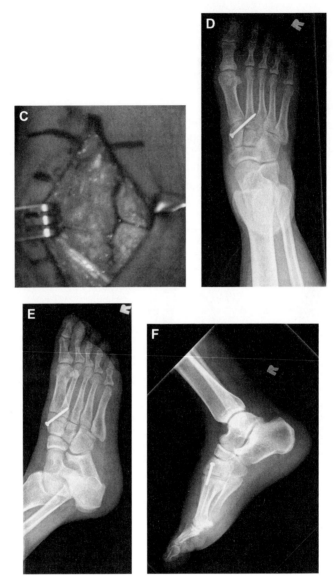

Fig. 1 (*continued*).

extensor hallucis longus and extensor hallucis brevis, which allows access to the medial–intermediate intercuneiform joint, the medial cuneiform–second metatarsal articulation, and the Lisfranc ligament. By dissecting superficial to the dorsalis pedis artery and deep peroneal nerve, the second TMT joint is exposed in the interval between the extensor hallucis brevis muscle and the extensor digitorum longus tendon to the second toe. The medial cuneiform–second metatarsal articulation and the Lisfranc ligament also can be exposed in this interval as can the third TMT joint. If needed, the incision can be extended proximally to access the naviculocuneiform joint. If needed, a second dorsal longitudinal incision is made overlying the fourth TMT joint or the interval between the third and fourth TMT joints. Taking care to avoid branches of the superficial peroneal nerve, the third, fourth, and fifth TMT joints can be exposed by dissecting between the extensor digitorum longus tendons and splitting the muscle belly of, or going between the tendons of, the extensor digitorum brevis.

The involved TMT joints are inspected to make sure that there is not excessive arthritis and that any interposed scar tissue and bone/cartilage fragments are removed. The second metatarsal medial cuneiform interval is exposed. Unlike the anterior talofibular or spring ligaments, the short length of the Lisfranc ligament and its location make imbrication difficult. Instead, excess tissue is removed from the medial second metatarsal base and the exposed bone is curetted to promote healing. A small incision is made over the medial aspect of the medial cuneiform. Reduction is obtained using a bone clamp between the medial aspect of the medial cuneiform and the lateral second metatarsal base, and is maintained with a 3.5-, 4-, or 4.5-mm screw. Although cannulated screws may be used, the author prefers to use intraoperative fluoroscopy and a cannulated 3.5-mm drill to make a gliding hole in the medial cuneiform and avoid the articular cartilage of the first TMT and medial–intermediate intercuneiform joints. The guide wire is removed, the second metatarsal base is drilled with a 2.5-mm drill, and a stronger and more cost-effective noncannulated 3.5-mm cortical lag screw is inserted. If desired, a cannulated drill can be used to make a tunnel dorsal to the screw for placement of a tendon graft to reconstruct the interosseous Lisfranc's ligament. Options for graft include autologous plantaris, peroneus tertius, extensor digitorum longus, or split anterior tibial tendons. Alternatively, allograft or synthetic materials may be used. The graft may be secured at the tunnel ends with suture or suture anchors or looped dorsally deep to the neurovascular structures and hallux extensor tendons and sutured back to itself. The dorsal TMT capsule and ligaments should be preserved and repaired if possible.

For subacute missed Lisfranc injuries that are limited mainly to subluxation of the second metatarsal, this generally is sufficient fixation. If there is residual instability at any of the other TMT, intercuneiform, or naviculocuneiform joints they can be stabilized with metallic or absorbable [31,35] intra-articular screws, k-wires, or bridging plates with the same advantages and disadvantages as for acute Lisfranc injuries. K-wires are best suited for temporary fixation of the more mobile fourth and fifth TMT joints. Screws provide stronger fixation than do k-wires, but cause additional intra-articular damage, and their often intra-articular distal threads are difficult to remove should the screw break. Plates have equivalent strength to screws and do not cause further articular damage, but may cause more soft tissue irritation [36].

Triceps surae contractures put increased dorsiflexion stress on the midfoot joints with gait. If there is less than neutral ankle dorsiflexion with the knee extended, the subtalar joint in neutral, and the TMT joints reduced, then strong consideration should be made for adding a gastrocnemius recession or an aggressive postoperative gastrocnemius/soleus stretching program.

Postoperative management after ORIF of nonacute Lisfranc joint injuries with or without Lisfranc ligament reconstruction is similar to acute injuries. The patient spends 6 weeks in a nonweight-bearing cast followed by 6 to 10 weeks of progressive weight-bearing in a CAM walker or orthotic. In athletes or reliable patients who undergo stable fixation, early motion and limited protected weight-bearing decreases muscle atrophy, disuse osteopenia, and joint stiffness.

The same controversies about hardware removal after ORIF of acute Lisfranc injuries apply to delayed reconstruction. Fixation across the fourth and fifth TMT joints is removed 6 to 12 weeks postoperatively to allow joint motion and prevent k-wire breakage. Fixation of the first, second, and third TMT joints should be left in place for at least 3 to 4 months to allow sufficient ligamentous healing. If removed earlier, there is an increased risk of recurrent TMT joint subluxation. Hardware removal allows TMT joint motion, addresses hardware-related soft tissue irritation, and eliminates the risk of intra-articular broken screws. However it requires the morbidity of a second operation, the medial three TMT joints' subsequent motion likely is minimal secondary to posttraumatic stiffness superimposed on its normal limited excursion, and there is the risk of recurrent subluxation if inadequate ligament healing has occurred.

Arthrodesis and arthroplasty

Arthrodesis is indicated for advanced arthritis or fixed or neuropathic deformity. Arthrodesis also may be considered over joint realignment and ligament reconstruction to reduce the risk of recurrent subluxation and progressive arthritis at the cost of loss of joint motion. If there is only malalignment at the second TMT joint an isolated arthrodesis of the second TMT and medial–intermediate intercuneiform joint may be performed through the same dorsomedial incision that is used for Lisfranc ligament reconstruction. Three screws, one from the medial cuneiform to the intermediate cuneiform, one from the medial cuneiform to the second metatarsal base, and one from the second metatarsal base to the intermediate cuneiform, are placed. Alternatively, dorsal plates, compression staples, and historically, dowel grafts may be used. If the third TMT is arthritic or remains unstable it may be fused with or without incorporating the intermediate–lateral intercuneiform joint. If the first TMT or naviculocuneiform joints are arthritic or have residual subluxation or deformity they also may be incorporated into the fusion mass. The naviculocuneiform joint can be accessed through the same dorsomedial incision or a medial longitudinal one. Arthrodesis should correct any preexisting deformity and restore the longitudinal arch. In these situations it is best to reduce and provisionally fix the first TMT and, if included, naviculocuneiform joints before the other TMT joints. Associated posterior tibial tendon dysfunction may be addressed concurrently with a posterior tibial tendon debridement or augmentation, a spring ligament repair, or a calcaneal osteotomy.

A significant triceps surae contracture is addressed with a gastrocnemius recession or Achilles tendon lengthening.

Mild to moderate fourth and fifth TMT joint arthritis often remains minimally symptomatic after fusion of the medial three TMT joints [19,37]. If there is significant fourth and fifth TMT joint arthritis, these joints also may be fused by way of the dorsolateral incision. Patients who have deformity and neuropathic arthritis of all five TMT joints may require a medial- and plantar-based closing wedge osteotomy through a medial longitudinal incision. Fixation can be obtained with crossed screws, a plantar-based first TMT plate [38], or external fixation. A resection arthroplasty that interposes a ceramic spacer or autologous tissue, such as the peroneus tertius or the extensor digitorum brevis, may be preferable to arthrodesis for the more mobile fourth and fifth TMT joints [39].

After arthrodesis, the patient is immobilized in a nonweight-bearing cast for 6 to 12 weeks until there is evidence of fusion; this is followed by progressive weight bearing in a CAM walker or orthotic.

Literature review and clinical decision making

Hardcastle and colleagues [17] noted only fair results in two patients who had Lisfranc joint injuries that were treated with open reduction and k-wire fixation more than 6 weeks after injury. They believed that it probably was better not to attempt reduction and fixation after 6 weeks from the date of injury. Faciszewski and colleagues [26] performed arthrodesis on two patients who presented at 4 months and 25 years after Lisfranc joint injury; the results were good and poor, respectively. One other patient was diagnosed 1 year after injury who they decided not to treat and had a fair outcome.

Chiodo and Myerson [15] have reduced TMT joint dislocations successfully with ORIF 1 year after injury. They stated that the success of such a late reduction depends upon the extent of articular incongruity and cannot be accomplished in the presence of a malunited fracture. Trevino and Kodros [29] stated that although good results have been obtained as late as 6 weeks after injury, the success of surgery after 6 weeks is diminished by multiple factors, including the need for extensive soft tissue dissection, destruction of articular surface because of malposition, and suboptimal stabilization of the Lisfranc ligament because of rounding of its edges.

Thordarson [40] believed that delayed ORIF could be performed; however, he stated that reduction is more difficult and may require indirect reduction techniques using an external fixator between the calcaneus and fifth metatarsal. He recommended placing one or two 3.5-mm cortical screws across all five TMT joints and leaving them in for a minimum of 6 months because of the higher likelihood of displacement as compared with acute fixation.

Davies and Saxby [5] treated three symptomatic patients who presented 2, 4, and 11 months after injury with gap signs between their hallux and second toes and intercuneiform widening. All patients had Lisfranc ligament ruptures observed intraoperatively. Screws were placed from the medial cuneiform into the intermediate cuneiform and second metatarsal base. A fusion was performed in the patient who presented 11 months out. In the other two patients the screws were placed to hold reduction until ligament healing occurred and were removed after 4 months. The toe diastasis resolved in all three patients. No clinical outcomes were given but one of the nonarthrodesed patients was pursuing a career as a ski instructor.

Kuo and colleagues [18] noted the presence of posttraumatic arthritis in 1 of 3 (33%) patients after ORIF of Lisfranc joint injuries after "delayed diagnosis" as compared with 11 of 45 (24%) patients after "acute diagnosis." Excluding patients who had contralateral lower extremity injuries, 2 patients with "delayed diagnosis" had an average American Orthopedic Foot and Ankle Society (AOFAS) midfoot score of 79, whereas 40 patients with "acute diagnosis" had an average AOFAS midfoot score of 80.2. The investigators noted a tendency for poorer results after acute ORIF for purely ligamentous Lisfranc injuries, including those with no fracture other than a small avulsion fracture at the Lisfranc ligament attachment site.

Allozo and colleagues [41] treated 10 patients who were diagnosed between 1 week and 36 months (average, 9 months) since injury with delayed reconstruction of the Lisfranc ligament. The scarred ligament was removed and reconstructed by way of drill holes using suture in 8 patients and using the extensor digitorum longus tendon to the fourth toe in the other 2 patients. At an average of 4 years of follow-up there were eight good results with no pain, weakness, or loss of anatomic reduction. Two patients had poor results; the initial reduction was suboptimal because of the presence of old fractures and stiffness of the soft issues and arthritis developed.

Thirteen patients who underwent ORIF more than 6 weeks (average 31.8 weeks) after Lisfranc joint injury were compared with 42 patients who had surgery within 6 weeks of injury at an average follow-up of 49.4 months. The group that had delayed diagnosis, all of whom had sustained pure ligamentous injuries without fracture, had a lower postoperative AOFAS midfoot score (64 versus 73.5) and a higher rate of subsequent midfoot arthrodesis (23% versus 9.5%) [42].

Calder and colleagues [43] noted 22 good (88%) and 3 (12%) poor results in patients who underwent ORIF within 3 months of sustaining a Lisfranc injury. Seventeen patients who underwent surgery more than 6 months after sustaining their injury were treated with primary fusion with 9 good (52.9%) and 8 (47.1%) poor results.

Several studies examined the results of midfoot arthrodesis for posttraumatic arthritis but did not separate out the results of patients whose Lisfranc injuries were missed initially, nor those who underwent arthrodesis as an index operation as opposed to those whose had undergone previous reduction and fixation [37,44,45]. Johnson and Johnson [44] noted satisfactory pain relief in 11 of 13 patients who underwent arthrodesis with dowel grafts. Sangeorzan and colleagues [37] noted 11 of 16 (69%) good or excellent results after fusion with lag screws. Mann and colleagues [45] found an average satisfaction index of 4 out of a possible 5 for 17 patients who underwent fusion of the TMT, intercuneiform, or naviculocuneiform joints.

Komenda and colleagues [46] reviewed 32 patients who underwent TMT arthrodesis for intractable pain after a traumatic midfoot injury; the diagnosis was missed initially in 10 patients and they had arthrodesis as their index procedure. The average time from injury to surgery was 34 months (range, 6–81 months) for the patients with missed injuries; their average AOFAS midfoot score increased from 41.1 to 82.2.

A recent prospective, randomized study evaluated 41 patients who had Lisfranc injuries that were treated within 3 months of injury by ORIF or primary arthrodesis of the medial two or three TMT joints [47]. At an average of 35 months of follow-up the 21 patients who underwent primary arthrodesis had a higher rate of return to preinjury level of activity (76% versus 55%) and a significantly higher mean AOFAS midfoot score (83 versus 62) than did the 20 patients who underwent ORIF.

Treatment recommendations

Lisfranc injuries that are at least 6 weeks old upon diagnosis, do not have associated fractures that require surgical stabilization, and do not meet radiographic criteria for significant TMT subluxation or instability are treated nonoperatively initially. Because first TMT joint hypermobility is not uncommon and often decreases secondary to postinjury scarring and immobilization, the author has a slightly higher threshold for sagittal plane motion of this joint in the absence of a history of symptomatic hallux valgus or lesser metatarsalgia. In the author's experience, patients who have preexisting cavovarus feet and metatarsus adductus seem better able to tolerate the slight increase in metatarsal abduction and dorsiflexion deformity that commonly are associated with mild TMT subluxation. If nonoperative treatment fails, arthrodesis of the symptomatic joints can be performed. Pain relief after diagnostic local anesthetic injections and radiographic evidence of arthritis and deformity help to determine which joints to arthrodese.

If there is significant TMT subluxation or instability with TMT joint arthritis then nonoperative treatment is recommended initially. If nonoperative treatment is unsuccessful, arthrodesis of any of the medial three TMTs or naviculocuneiform joints that are symptomatic is recommended. In the absence of severe and markedly symptomatic arthritis, the fourth and fifth TMTs may be left intact. If the fourth and fifth TMT joints continue to be symptomatic or if they have severe arthritis a fusion or resection arthroplasty may be performed. Arthroplasty is recommended in younger, more active individuals. Fourth and fifth TMT arthrodesis is preferable for neuropathic arthropathy.

If there is TMT subluxation or instability in the absence of arthritis, open reduction and rigid internal fixation is recommended to decrease the risk of subsequent arthritis, particularly if there is just mild subluxation of only the medial–intermediate intercuneiform joint or second TMT joint. In more extensive Lisfranc joint dislocations—particularly pure ligamentous ones, those in patients who have neuropathy, and possibly all unstable if displaced Lisfranc injuries, primary arthrodesis may be more appropriate. If primary arthrodesis would be the surgeon's choice for a given clinical scenario, an initial trial of conservative treatment with arthrodesis as a salvage procedure may be considered particularly in an elderly, low demand patient.

Summary

Lisfranc injuries, particularly subtle low-energy ones, may be missed at the time of injury and can leave the patient with persistent instability, deformity, and/or arthritis. In the presence of neuropathic arthropathy, significant residual arthritis, or fixed deformity that is recalcitrant to conservative treatment, arthrodesis, including correction of deformity, is the treatment of choice for the first, second, and third TMT joints. Usually, fourth and fifth TMT joints are treated by observation or resection arthroplasty unless neuropathic. In the absence of residual arthritis or fixed deformity, delayed ORIF with or without reconstruction of Lisfranc's ligament may be performed. An alternative is reduction and primary arthrodesis of the involved medial TMT joints.

References

[1] Kura H, Luo Z, Kitaoka H, et al. Mechanical behavior of the Lisfranc and dorsal cuneometatarsal ligaments: in vitro biomechanical study. J Orthop Trauma 2001;15:107–10.

[2] Solan M, Moorman III C, Miyamoto RG, et al. Ligamentous restraints of the second tarsometatarsal joint: a biomechanical evaluation. Foot Ankle Int 2001;22:637–41.

[3] Ouzounian T, Shereff MJ. In vitro determination of midfoot motion. Foot Ankle 1989;10:140–6.

[4] Ross G, Cronin R, Hauzenblas J, et al. Plantar ecchymosis sign: a clinical aid to diagnosis of occult Lisfranc tarsometatarsal injuries. J Orthop Trauma 1996;10:119–22.

[5] Davies MS, Saxby TS. Intercuneiform instability and the "gap" sign. Foot Ankle Int 1999;20: 606–29.

[6] Peicha G, Preidler KW, Lajtai G, et al. Diagnostic value of conventional roentgen image, computerized and magnetic resonance tomography in acute sprains of the foot. A prospective clinical study. Unfallchirurg 2001;104:1134–9.

[7] Lu J, Ebraheim NA, Skie M, et al. Radiographic and computed tomographic evaluation of Lisfranc dislocation: a cadaver study. Foot Ankle Int 1997;18:351–5.

[8] Brunet JA, Wiley JJ. The late results of tarsalmetatarsal joint injuries. J Bone Joint Surg 1987; 69-B:437–40.

[9] Aitken AP, Poulson D. Dislocations of the tarsometatarsal joint. J Bone Joint Surg 1963;45-A: 246–60.

[10] Arntz CT, Hansen ST. Dislocations and fracture dislocations of the tarsometatarsal joints. Orthop Clin North Am 1987;18:105–14.

[11] Arntz CT, Veith RG, Hansen ST. Fractures and fracture-dislocations of the tarsometatarsal joint. J Bone Joint Surg 1988;70A:173–81.

[12] Bloome DM, Clanton TO. Treatment of Lisfranc injuries in the athlete. Tech Foot Ankle Surg 2002;1:94–101.

[13] Buzzard BM, Briggs PJ. Surgical management of acute tarsometatarsal fracture dislocation in the adult. Clin Orthop 1998;353:125–33.

[14] Cassebaum WH. Lisfrance fracture-dislocations. Clin Orthop 1964;30:116–28.

[15] Chiodo C, Myerson M. Developments and advances in the diagnosis and treatment of injuries to the tarsometatarsal joint. Orthop Clin North Am 2001;32:11–20.

[16] Goossens M, DeStoop N. Lisfranc's fracture-dislocations: etiology, radiology, and results of treatment. Clin Orthop 1983;176:154–62.

[17] Hardcastle PH, Reschauer R, Kutscha-Lissberg E, et al. Injuries to the tarsometatarsal joint. J Bone Joint Surg 1982;64-B:349–56.

[18] Kuo R, Tejwani N, DiGiovanni CW, et al. Outcome after open reduction and internal fixation of Lisfranc joint injuries. J Bone Joint Surg 2000;82-A:1609–18.

[19] Myerson MS. The diagnosis and treatment of injury to the tarsometatarsal joint complex. J Bone Joint Surg 2001;81B:756–63.

[20] Myerson MS, Fisher RT, Burgess AR, et al. Fracture dislocations of the tarsometatarsal joints: end results correlated with pathology and treatment. Foot Ankle 1986;6:225–42.

[21] Resch S, Stenstrom A. The treatment of tarsometatarsal injuries. Foot Ankle 1990;11:117–23.

[22] Rutledge EW, Templeman DC, deSouza LJ. Evaluation and treatment of Lisfranc fracture-dislocations. Foot Ankle Clin 1999;4:603–15.

[23] Schenk Jr RC, Heckman JD. Fractures and dislocations of the forefoot: operative and non-operative treatment. J Am Acad Orthop Surg 1995;3:70–8.

[24] Wilppula E. Tarsometatarsal fracture-dislocation: late results in 26 patients. Acta Orthop Scand 1973;44:335–45.

[25] Wiss DA, Kull DM, Perry J. Lisfranc fracture-dislocations of the foot: a clinical-kinesiological study. J Orthop Trauma 1988;1:267–74.

[26] Faciszewski T, Burks R, Manaster BJ. Subtle injuries of the Lisfranc joint. J Bone Joint Surg 1990;72A:1519–22.

[27] Potter H, Deland JT, Gusmer PB, et al. Magnetic resonance imaging of the Lisfranc ligament of the foot. Foot Ankle Int 1998;19:438–45.

[28] Teng AL, Pinzur MS, Lomasney L, et al. Functional outcome following anatomic restoration of tarsal-metatarsal fracture dislocation. Foot Ankle Int 2002;23:922–6.

[29] Trevino SG, Kodros S. Controversies in tarsometatarsal joints. Orthop Clin North Am 1995; 26:229–38.

[30] Stein RE. Radiological aspects of the tarsometatarsal joints. Foot Ankle 1983;3:286–9.

[31] Thordarson DB. Lisfranc ORIF with absorbable fixation. Tech Foot Ankle Surg 2003;2:21–6.

[32] Ebraheim NA, Yang H, Lu J, et al. Computer evaluation of second tarsometatarsal joint dislocation. Foot Ankle Int 1996;17:685–9.

[33] Coss H, Manos RE, Buoncristiani A, et al. Abduction stress and AP weightbearing radiography of purely ligamentous injury in the tarsometatarsal joint. Foot Ankle Int 1998;19: 538–41.

[34] Lakin RC, DeGnore LT, Pienkowski D. Contact mechanics of normal tarsometatarsal joints. J Bone Joint Surg 2001;83A:520–8.

[35] Thordarson DB, Hurwitz G. PLA screw fixation of Lisfranc injuries. Foot Ankle Int 2003;23: 1003–7.

[36] Alberta F, Aronow MS, Barrero M, et al. Ligamentous Lisfranc joint injuries: a biomechanical comparison of dorsal plate and trans-articular screw fixation. Foot Ankle Int 2005;26:462–73.

[37] Sangeorzan BJ, Veith R, Hansen ST. Salvage of Lisfranc's tarsometatarsal joint by arthrodesis. Foot Ankle Int 1990;10:193–200.

[38] Marks R, Parks B, Schon LC. Midfoot fusion technique for neuroarthropathic feet: biomechanical analysis and rationale. Foot Ankle Int 1998;19:507–10.

[39] Berlet GC, Anderson RB. Tendon arthroplasty for basal fourth and fifth metatarsal arthritis. Foot Ankle Int 2002;23:440–6.

[40] Thordarson DB. Fractures of the midfoot and forefoot. In: Myerson MS, editor. Foot and ankle disorders. Philadelphia: W.B. Saunders Company; 2000. p. 1277–8.

[41] Alloza JFM, Nery C, Barroco R, et al. Subtle lesions of the intercuneiform and tarsometatarsal

joints treated by neoligament plasty. Presented at the International Federation of Foot and Ankle Societies Triennial Scientific Meeting. San Francisco, September 14, 2002.

[42] Philbin T, Rosenberg G, Sferra JJ. Complications of missed or untreated Lisfranc injuries. Foot Ankle Clin 2003;8:61–71.

[43] Calder JDF, Whitehouse SL, Saxby TS. Results of isolated Lisfranc injuries and the effect of compensation claims. J Bone Joint Surg Br 2004;86:527–30.

[44] Johnson JE, Johnson KA. Dowel arthrodesis for degenerative arthritis of the tarsometatarsal (Lisfranc) joints. Foot Ankle 1986;6:243–53.

[45] Mann RA, Prieskorn D, Sobel M. Mid-tarsal and tarsometatarsal arthrodesis for primary degenerative osteoarthrosis or osteoarthrosis after trauma. J Bone Joint Surg Am 1996;78:1376–85.

[46] Komenda GA, Myerson MS, Biddinger KR. Results of arthrodesis of the tarsometatarsal joints after traumatic injury. J Bone Joint Surg Am 1996;78:1665–76.

[47] Ly TV, Coetzee CJ. Treatment of ligamentous Lisfranc injuries: primary arthrodesis vs. ORIF. Presented at the 35th Annual Winter Meeting of the American Orthopaedic Foot and Ankle Society Washington, DC, February 26, 2005.

ELSEVIER
SAUNDERS

Foot Ankle Clin N Am
11 (2006) 143–163

FOOT AND
ANKLE CLINICS

First Ray Injuries

John D. Maskill, MD[a],*, Donald R. Bohay, MD[b,c],
John G. Anderson, MD[b,c]

[a]*Grand Rapids Medical Education and Research Center/Michigan State University,
Orthopaedic Surgery Residency Program, 300 Lafayette, Grand Rapids, MI 49503, USA*
[b]*Department of Orthopaedic Surgery, College of Human Medicine,
Michigan State University, MI, USA*
[c]*Orthopaedic Associates of Grand Rapids P.C., Foot and Ankle Division, 1111 Leffingwell NE,
Suite 100, Grand Rapids, MI 49525, USA*

Fractures of the forefoot are common and can lead to significant pain and prolonged disability and dysfunction. These injuries can result in malunion, non-union, and joint stiffness. Difficulties with ambulation and abnormalities of load distribution may occur.

The forefoot serves two purposes during gait. As a unit, it provides a broad plantar surface on which to share the weight of the body. Weight-bearing studies showed that the two sesamoids and the four lesser metatarsal heads share an equal amount of the forefoot load in normal gait [1]. Secondly, the forefoot is structured to be mobile in the sagittal plane. This mobility provides the forefoot with the ability to alter the position of the metatarsal heads in space so as to accommodate uneven ground, which allows the foot to maintain an even pressure distribution on its plantar surface. Although the forefoot appears to work as a single unit, its parts are distinctly different and should be treated accordingly in case of injury.

This article addresses first ray injuries specifically. The first ray differs from the other rays in its position and its importance with weight bearing; the tripod stance of the foot is formed with the fifth ray and the calcaneus. Injuries to the first ray can cause critical alterations in the biomechanics of the foot, which allow for pathologic weight-bearing points of contact and deformity that lead to a disabling gait.

* Corresponding author.
  E-mail address: djmaskill@comcast.net (J.D. Maskill).

1083-7515/06/$ – see front matter © 2006 Elsevier Inc. All rights reserved.
doi:10.1016/j.fcl.2005.12.002   *foot.theclinics.com*

Physicians who are involved in the care of the foot and ankle, especially in athletes, must be familiar with the spectrum of injuries concerning the first ray, the nonoperative and operative treatment options, and the concurrent sequelae that follow if they are not managed appropriately.

First metatarsal fractures

Anatomy

The first metatarsocuneiform joint is formed by the trapezoidal base of the first metatarsal and the anterior articular surface of the medial cuneiform. The anterior surface of the medial cuneiform is slightly convex in the transverse plane and is nearly flat in the vertical plane. Some variation exists in the medial inclination of the joint in the transverse plane; the normal range is between 8° and 10° [2].

In general, stability of the tarsometatarsal joint complex is created by its bony architecture. The base of the second metatarsal is recessed and forms a keylike configuration with the middle cuneiform that restricts motion and imparts rigidity to the second ray. The trapezoidal shape of all of the metatarsal bases forms a "Roman arch" configuration, which prevents plantar displacement of the metatarsals [3–5].

To augment the osseous architecture, the Lisfranc ligament runs between the medial cuneiform and the base of the second metatarsal, which further increases the stability of the second tarsometatarsal joint. The other four metatarsal bases are joined together by a strong ligament; however, no similar structure exists between the first metatarsal and the lateral four metatarsals. This allows for independent motion. Strong thick ligaments that make up the capsule of the first tarsometatarsal joint support its resting position [3–5].

The first metatarsal also is unique in its configuration. It is shorter and wider than the lesser four metatarsals. The anterior tibialis inserts onto the plantarmedial aspect of the first metatarsal base, and the peroneus longus attaches onto the plantarlateral base of the first metatarsal. These two muscles serve to position the first metatarsal head in space; the anterior tibialis elevates the head, and the peroneus longus plantarflexes the head. Although mechanisms for plantarflexion and dorsiflexion operate through the first tarsometatarsal joint, motion is limited in normal feet [6]. The first metatarsal head supports two sesamoids bones, which provide two of the six contact points of the forefoot. Therefore, the first ray essentially supports at least one third of the forefoot weight at any given time [1,6].

Mechanism of injury

First metatarsal fractures can result from direct and indirect forces. Direct forces that result in crush injuries are common in industry [6,7]. In addition to the first metatarsal, the soft tissues take a large portion of the impact, which causes many of these to be open fractures [6]. Twisting injuries occur when the foot is fixed on the ground and the patient turns, which creates torque on the metatarsal, and thus, causes a fracture. An axial load also may cause a fracture. In this case, the first metatarsal is impacted into the medial cuneiform. The first tarsometatarsal joint can become stressed and later attenuated as it sometimes takes most of the force (see later discussion). Because of the tendinous insertions, avulsion fractures can occur with plantarflexion and inversion-type injuries.

Clinical diagnosis

The importance of investigating the history and intensity of the trauma that produced the fracture cannot be overemphasized. Given the innate structure of the first metatarsal, a significant amount of force usually is required to cause a fracture. Giannestras and Sammarco [8] cautioned against casually reducing a first metatarsal fracture and treating it closed in a cast. The potential is great for skin slough that involves a large area of the dorsum of the foot in a traumatic injury. Soft tissue damage can be devastating and should be the first priority [2,6–8]. After the soft tissue has been assessed, a thorough neurovascular examination should be performed.

Clinically, patients usually experience pain over the first metatarsal and are unable to bear weight. Typically, the foot is swollen and ecchymotic over the first ray. Pain, motion, and crepitance can be produced with flexion and extension of the distal fragment. If an impaction injury is suspected, axial pressure may reproduce pain in the metatarsal [9].

Radiographic assessment

Routine anteroposterior (AP), oblique, and lateral radiographs of the foot should be obtained if a fracture is suspected. The fracture should be visualized on at least two views. Often, the AP and oblique views are most helpful because the metatarsals are overlapped on the lateral view; however, the lateral view reveals dorsal or plantar displacement of the fracture fragments. Weight-bearing stress views should be done if possible to determine stability of the fracture. First metatarsal base fractures may require a CT scan, if suspicion is high enough, to evaluate better the fragment size and the integrity of the first metatarsocuneiform joint [2]. Bone scans can be used to detect a stress fracture.

Treatment

Significant forces exist through the first metatarsal during gait; therefore, it is important to maintain its position in the normal cascade of the forefoot. The criteria for intervention are based on the stability of the fracture and the adjacent joint. There are no ligamentous supports from this metatarsal to adjacent structures, so any fracture displacement is likely to represent an unstable fracture pattern.

Instability can be determined by way of stress radiographs if a fracture pattern is displaced minimally. Any displacement of the fracture or displacement through the joint with manual stress is perceived as instability [10]. If no instability is noted on stress views, and no other injury of the midfoot or metatarsals exists, isolated, stable first metatarsal fractures can be treated in a short leg cast. Weight-bearing status varies by surgeon. LaPorta [11] preferred a short leg cast, with no weight bearing for 6 weeks, followed by a rigid-soled shoe for several additional weeks. Garcia and Parks [9] and Giannestras and Sammarco [8] recommended treating patients in a short leg cast, with no weight bearing for 2 to 3 weeks, followed by a walking cast for an additional 3 weeks. Mann and Coughlin [12] preferred a well-molded cast with weight bearing starting on day 7 to 10. The cast is removed when radiographic evidence of healing is present and the patient is placed into a stiff-soled shoe. When casting this type of injury, it is important to position the foot in a plantigrade position without placing dorsally or plantarly directed pressure on the first metatarsal. This could lead to malunion if the first ray is plantarflexed or dorsiflexed thus producing alterations in the weight-bearing pattern of the forefoot [9,10].

If instability is present, the fracture should be treated aggressively with surgical stabilization. The goals of internal fixation are to restore the normal anatomic features of the first metatarsal, the sesamoids, and the first meta-tarsophalangeal (MTP) joint.

Simple fractures, whether diaphyseal or intra-articular, are treated best with lag screw fixation with 2.7-mm screws after open reduction. A supplemental neutralization plate could be added for increased stability of the construct. After the fracture has been stabilized, reassessment of the first tarsometatarsal joint needs to be performed. If the joint is unstable, a 3.5-mm cortical screw is placed both distal–proximal and proximal–distal to stabilize the joint. This is similar to the construct that is used for a Lisfranc injury. If the fracture configuration does not allow this type of construct, a one-third tubular bridging plate could be used, which extends from the medial cuneiform to the first metatarsal. To protect the extensor tendons, plates can be applied to the medial side of the metatarsal [6]. Ultimately, the soft tissue should dictate where the plate is placed to minimize the amount of disruption.

When lag screw fixation is not feasible, based on the extent of the comminution, a bridging plate also could be used solely on the first metatarsal; the determining factor is whether adequate proximal and distal fixation exists. If severe comminution is the case with inadequate bone to support a plate, then external fixation is the treatment of choice. The surgeon's goal is to maintain length of the first metatarsal to prevent transfer lesions from occurring under the lateral lesser metatarsal heads. Often, injuries with extensive comminution also have a significant soft tissue component. External fixation also is minimally invasive, which makes the technique a wise choice for the management of these fractures.

In using an external fixator on the first ray, if the proximal phalanx is used in the construct, care should be taken to ensure that the foot remains in a plantigrade position. The proximal phalanx should be dorsiflexed slightly if possible to prevent problems of toe position in the event of a stiff joint after injury [10].

Fractures of the metatarsal head should be treated in an attempt to preserve articular function. If displacement and disruption of the articular surface is present, the fracture should be opened and stabilized. Cancellous bone graft can be used behind the subchondral bone for support if needed. Anatomic reduction should be the goal. Large intra-articular fracture fragments can be held with smooth k-wires or miniscrews. In the presence of comminution of the head or neck an external fixator can be used to maintain length by way of ligamentotaxis. The fixator should incorporate the proximal phalanx [10].

Postoperative care

Postoperatively, the soft tissues determine the type of immobilization that is warranted. If the soft tissues are reasonable, a short leg cast is appropriate. The patient should be kept nonweight bearing for 6 to 8 weeks and then transferred into a postoperative boot/shoe. In the boot, range of motion of the great toe is encouraged if this was not incorporated originally into the construct.

In the presence of an external fixator, a removable molded splint should be used to maintain a plantigrade position. After the bridging callus is identified, the fixator can be removed and the foot can be placed into a postoperative boot. The patient can start to bear weight as tolerated. After 10 weeks the patient can wean himself/herself into a normal shoe. Progression of activity is based on patient comfort.

Complications

Malunion, nonunion, and posttraumatic arthrosis of the tarsometatarsal or MTP joints are possible. This is based on the effectiveness of the fixation or lack thereof.

If the first metatarsal is short or not plantigrade then transfer lesions will occur from excessive weight bearing of the lesser metatarsal heads. Ultimately, this could result in MTP synovitis and then a rupture of the plantar plate or collateral ligaments that culminate in a hammer toe deformity or a cross-over toe deformity, respectively (Fig. 1).

In occult injuries to the metatarsocuneiform joint, a traumatic bunion can occur. This is secondary to the attenuation of the capsuloligamentous structures of the first tarsometatarsal joint. Keep in mind the minimal restraints to the first ray at this level in the foot. The bunion is caused by medial angulation of the first metatarsal that results in hallux valgus. This situation allows for a hypermobile, dynamically elevated first ray that leads to transfer lesions and various toe deformities [3]. One must have a high suspicion of this lesion to diagnose it, because it is reportedly missed in as many as 20% of cases [3]. Treatment is fusion of the first tarsometatarsal joint in a plantigrade position.

First metatarsophalangeal joint injuries

Since the term "turf toe" was first termed in the literature by Bowers and Martin [13] in 1976, injuries to the hallux MTP joint have received increased

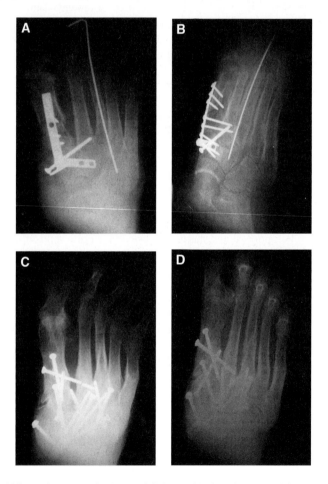

Fig. 1. A middle-aged man sustained a crush injury to his foot that resulted in severe soft tissue disruption as well as a Lisfranc injury and first metatarsal fracture with severe comminution. (A, B) A bridging plate was used initially with the midfoot lag screw fixation technique. (C–E) The patient went on to a nonunion and underwent a revision open reduction with internal fixation; however, the first metatarsal was severely short after surgery. The patient went on to develop midfoot arthritis and multiple transfer lesions across the metatarsal pad with severe hammer toe deformities. (F, G) The patient underwent metatarsal shortening osteotomies with hammer toe corrections in an attempt to alleviate symptoms.

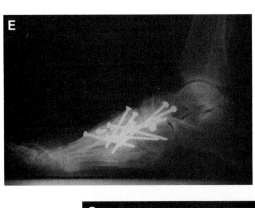

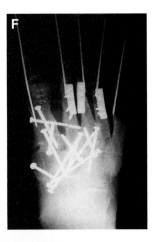

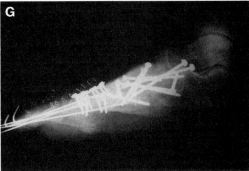

Fig. 1 (*continued*).

attention from physicians, trainers, and athletes. Several collegiate and professional athletes with a variety of soft tissue injuries to the hallux MTP joint have been seen. Historically, these injuries have been grouped under the general heading of "turf toe," but they represent a broad spectrum of severity.

Anatomy

The MTP joint of the hallux allows for plantarflexion and dorsiflexion primarily. Adduction and abduction are limited. Motion of this joint consists of rolling, sliding, and compression. More than one center of motion is present, which makes it like a hammock or dynamic acetabulum as described by Kelikian [14,15]. The joint articulation provides little of the overall stability because of the shallow glenoidlike cavity of the proximal phalanx. Most of this stability comes from the surrounding capsuloligamentous–sesamoid complex.

Two sets of ligaments contribute to the stability of the hallux MTP joint: the medial and lateral collateral ligaments and the medial and lateral metatarsosesamoid suspensory ligaments (Fig. 2). In addition to these ligaments, the strong,

A   **B**

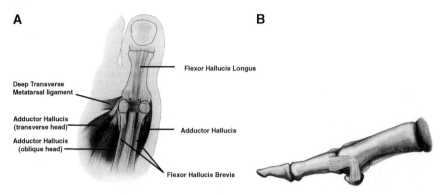

Fig. 2. Applied anatomy of the first MTP joint. (*A*) Dorsal view of the plantar structures of the first MTP joint. (*B*) View of the collateral ligamentous attachments of the first MTP joint. (*From* Early JS. Fractures and dislocations of the midfoot and forefoot. In: Bucholz, Heckman, editors. Rockwood and Green's Fractures in Adults. 5th edition. Lippincott Williams and Wilkins; 2001. p. 2229.)

fibrous plantar plate affords significant support. This plantar plate is attached firmly to the base of the proximal phalanx and is attached only loosely at the metatarsal neck through the capsule.

The tendon of the flexor hallucis brevis runs along the plantar aspect of the hallux, splits, and envelopes the sesamoids just before the two heads insert into the base of the proximal phalanx. A thick intersesamoid ligament unites the two sesamoids. This helps to maintain the course of the flexor hallucis longus tendon. The abductor and adductor hallucis tendons insert on the medial and lateral aspects of the hallux MTP, respectively. The capsuloligamentous complex of the first MTP joint is a confluence of structures that includes the collateral ligaments, plantar plate, the flexor hallucis brevis, the adductor hallucis, and the abductor hallucis tendons (see Fig. 2).

The extensor hallucis brevis originates with the extensor digitorum brevis at the calcaneus and runs obliquely across the dorsum of the foot to insert into the extensor mechanism of the first MTP joint.

Biomechanics

During normal gait, the great toe typically supports twice the load of the lesser toes and accommodates forces that reach 40% to 60% of body weight [16]. During athletic activities peak forces are even higher, and approach two to three times body weight with jogging and running, and eight times body weight with a running jump [17].

The range of motion in the normal foot has been studied extensively. In the resting position, the hallux MTP joint is in a mean position of 16° of dorsiflexion. The passive arc of motion was noted by Joseph [18] to be from 3° to 43° of plantarflexion and from 40° to 100° of dorsiflexion. The mean passive MTP joint dorsiflexion in normal gait during push-off was 84°. Bojsen-Miller and Lamoreux

[19] found that at least 60° of dorsiflexion is considered normal in barefoot walking on a level surface. Athletes have been shown to be able to accommodate for up to 50% reduction in MTP joint motion by various gait adjustments, such as foot and leg external rotation, shortened stride, and increased ankle, knee, or hip motion [20]. In addition, a well-constructed, stiff-soled shoe is capable of decreasing MTP joint dorsiflexion to 25° to 30° without affecting gait significantly [19].

Mechanism of injury

When an athlete rises on the ball of the foot for activities, such as initiating a jump, or while running, the hallux MTP joint extends to approximately 100° (Fig. 3). As the proximal phalanx extends, the sesamoids are pulled distally and the dorsal portion of the metatarsal head articular surface bears most of the load. When an axial load is placed on the heel with the foot fixed in equinus, the plantar complex of the first MTP attenuates or ruptures and the unrestricted dorsiflexion can cause an impaction of the proximal phalanx on the dorsal metatarsal head. This mechanism leads to a broad spectrum of injuries that ranges from sprains of the plantar structures to frank dislocation [14].

Additionally, it is believed that the artificial surface on which the athletes play may be partly responsible for some of the injuries. Rodeo and colleagues [21] studied 80 professional football players and noted that 83% of those who sustained a turf toe injury did so on artificial turf. Nigg and Segesser [22] demonstrated an increased incidence of hallux MTP injures on artificial turf and attributed this to the enhanced friction that is inherent in the surface. This may

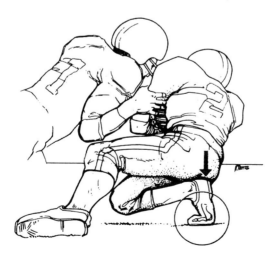

Fig. 3. "Turf toe" typically occurs when the first MTP joint is hyperextended. Additional trauma can occur if an axial load is then applied to the heel. (*From* Rodeo SA, O'Brien S, Warren RF. Turf-toe: an analysis of metatarsophalangeal joint sprains in professional football players. Am J Sports Med 1990;18:284; with permission.)

account for the forefoot becoming fixed to the artificial surface with applied external forces causing hyperextension and resulting in injury.

Bowers and Martin [13] and Clanton [23] commented on the idea that the shoe–surface interface could be responsible for these injuries. Most injuries are encountered on artificial turf in athletes who are wearing flexible soccer-style shoes. Athletes have abandoned the traditional heavier grass shoe with the steel plate incorporated into it for cleat attachment. During the 25 years before 1986, the trainers and physicians for Rice University could not recall a single instance of a severe MTP joint sprain occurring in a football player who wore the traditional grass shoe [24].

Not all injuries to the first MTP joint are due to hyperextension. Varus and valgus stresses to the joint also can cause injury and result in deformity [25–27]. These injuries are rare. Douglas and colleagues [25] reported on a soccer player who sustained a medial-sided injury from a valgus stress. He failed conservative therapy, developed a traumatic bunion deformity, and continued to complain of joint instability and pain; the medial ligaments were repaired [20]. Mullis and Miller [26] reported on a basketball player who sustained an injury to the lateral side of the MTP joint. He did not have deformity; however, he had difficulty running and was unable to return to sport. His injury was repaired and it was noted that all plantar structures were intact and only the lateral structures were torn.

Hyperflexion is the final mechanism that is noted with injuries to the hallux MTP joint. Some consider this sprain to be a variation of turf toe [27]. Frey and colleagues [28] coined the term "sand toe" because they noted that this injury was common in beach volleyball players. Rodeo and colleagues [21] also noted that hyperflexion injuries were present among football players. They found that 85% of "turf toe" injuries occurred with dorsiflexion and 12% occurred with plantarflexion. Watson and colleagues [14] saw this entity among classical and modern dancers.

Diagnosis

Diagnosis of a first MTP joint injury requires suspicion on the part of the examiner. Pain with weight bearing or exertional activities may be the only clue to an isolated mild injury. Ecchymosis and swelling are not always present initially. The loss of the normal parabolic cascade also is evidence of possible injury. Close palpation of the joint should be performed to discern the structures that are involved. The presence of active and passive stability of the joint as well as the range of joint motion in all planes should be assessed and compared with the contralateral foot. Instability in any plane denotes a significant injury [10,14]. A useful tool in assessing the stability of the joint is the dorsoplantar translation test. Any asymmetry, or increased translation, relative to the contralateral side denotes significant instability of the capsuloligamentous complex [29].

Radiographs also are important while assessing the first MTP joint complex. Weight-bearing AP and lateral films should be taken of the forefoot. Medial and lateral oblique views along with a sesamoid view also can be helpful. The injured foot always should be compared radiographically with the uninjured side.

Radiographs could reveal intra-articular fractures that may show a significant step-off. Avulsion fractures often are a clue that a collateral ligament or tendon has pulled off its insertion. The sesamoid position relative to each other as well as to the proximal phalanx also should be assessed and compared with the uninjured side. On the AP view, the distance between the base of the proximal phalanx to the distal pole of either sesamoid should be within 3 mm of the sesamoid position on the contralateral foot. If a partite sesamoid is present, the normal distance between the proximal phalangeal base and the distal pole of the sesamoid should be less than 10 mm for the tibial sesamoid and 13 mm for the fibular sesamoid. Distances greater than this denote plantar plate disruption 99% of the time [13].

Classification

Sprains or nondislocated injuries have been classified into grades I, II, and III based on the clinical examination (Box 1). Treatment and outcome correlate well with the initial grade [10]. Dislocations were classified initially by Jahss and were modified as other variations were noted. In general, type I dislocations involve an intact plantar plate (Fig. 4). Type II dislocations involve a partial disruption of the plantar plate. Type III dislocations have complete disruption of the plantar plate from the proximal phalanx (Fig. 5).

Treatment

Treatment of all grades of sprain/strain of the first MTP joint (turf toe, sand toe) are similar in the early stages. Clanton and colleagues [24,27] and Frey and colleagues [28] suggested using rest, ice, compression, and elevation. In some cases the joint may need to be immobilized. This can be accomplished with the use of a walker boot or a short leg cast, which includes a toe spica. In the spica, the toe is plantarflexed mildly to reduce the stretch on the plantar structures. Early joint motion can start within 3 to 5 days as symptoms allow [27,28]. Depending on the grade of the injury, the athlete can be advised about his return to sport and the necessary time for rehabilitation.

Athletes who have a grade I injury often can return to sport with little or no loss of playing time. These patients may benefit from taping the great toe to the lateral two toes for comfort. The taping is designed to decrease the amount of dorsiflexion or plantarflexion that the patient experiences. Another method that is used to reduce joint motion is the use of a stiff shoe. An insole that includes a spring carbon fiber steel plate in the forefoot region reduces the amount of motion at the first MTP joint.

Grade II injuries usually result in a loss of playing time that ranges from 3 to 14 days. The same treatment modalities are used as with the grade I injuries. Grade III injuries, however, often result in approximately 4 to 6 weeks of lost playing time. Most often, these patients require long-term immobilization

---

Box 1. First metatarsophalangeal joint injuries

Hyperextension injury (turf toe)

Grade I: stretching of the capsuloligamentous complex

Grade II: tear of capsular structures, without articular damage

Grade III: tear of capsular structures; articular compression
              injury dorsally
              Associated injury include
              • medial/lateral injury
              • sesamoid fracture
              • diastasis of sesamoids

Hyperflexion injury (sand toe)
Tear or sprain of the dorsal capsular structures

Dislocation

Type I: dislocation of the hallux with the sesamoids
              • No disruption of the intersesamoid ligament
              • Usually irreducible

Type IIA: dislocation with longitudinal disruption of the
              plantar plate and intersesamoid ligament

Type IIB: dislocation with partial disruption of the plantar
              plate with disruption of medial or lateral sesamoid

Type IIIA: dislocation with complete soft tissue disruption of
              the plantar complex from the proximal phalanx

Type IIIB: dislocation with complete plantar plate disruption,
              including disruption of one sesamoid

---

of the joint. Patients who experience persistent pain may benefit from physical therapy with other modalities, such as ultrasound with cold compression and whirlpool. The patient may return to play when the symptoms abate. This usually coincides with a painless passive range of motion of 50° to 60° [14,29].

Operative intervention for a turf toe or sand toe injury is indicated rarely, except in cases of intra-articular fractures or significant instability or deformity [20]. Avulsion fragments that are associated with a traumatic bunion deformity might need to be addressed by open reduction and ligamentous repair [29]. Dis-

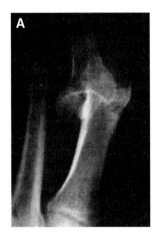
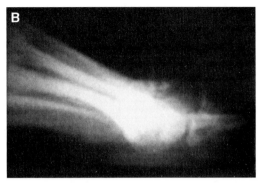

Fig. 4. AP (*A*) and lateral (*B*) views of an irreducible type I dislocation of the first MTP joint.

placed intra-articular fractures or osteochondral lesions should be fixed or debrided depending on their size and the amount of step-off.

Reported experience in the literature regarding dislocations of the first MTP joint is lacking. It seems that all investigators agree that acute dislocations should be reduced promptly to minimize any further soft tissue damage. Initial reduction can be done manually or with finger traps attached to the toe suspending the heel off the ground. An easy reduction usually is a clue that significant damage has been done to the plantar plate. It often means that there is no inherent stability after the joint is reduced [30–33]. If the plantar plate is intact, the initial dislocation usually is not reducible by closed means. If the dislocation is associated with fractures or disruption of the first tarsometatarsal

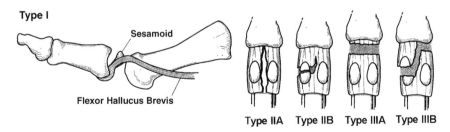

Fig. 5. Modified Jahss first MTP dislocation classification. Type I: the plantar plate and intersesamoid ligament are intact and dorsally displaced on the first metatarsal head. Often, open reduction is required. Type IIA: the plantar plate sustains a longitudinal split. The sesamoids are wide and often it is difficult to perform a closed reduction. Type IIB: the plantar plate is ruptured partially with a concomitant sesamoid fracture. This is amenable to closed reduction. Type IIIA: complete soft tissue disruption of the plantar plate from the proximal phalanx. The sesamoids are proximal on radiographs. Type IIIB: complete disruption of the plantar plate associated with a sesamoid fracture. (*From* Early JS. Fractures and dislocations of the midfoot and forefoot. In: Bucholz, Heckman, editors. Rockwood and Green's Fractures in Adults. 5th edition. Lippincott Williams and Wilkins; 2001. p. 2231).

joint, reductions can be possible. In these cases, the reduction should be done before the proximal lesion is stabilized [10]. Many of these dislocations that occur as the result of high-energy trauma have plantar wounds that may need debridement [30].

In the presence of an irreducible joint or gross instability, operative intervention becomes necessary to restore stability and function. The irreducible joint is usually due to the intact plantar plate resting dorsal to the metatarsal head (Jahss type I). An irreducible joint also can be seen if the plantar plate splits longitudinally and the metatarsal head buttonholes through the plantar plate (Jahss type IIA). These two types of dislocations can be differentiated by radiographs. The sesamoids are together in a type I injury, whereas they are divergent in a type IIA injury. Typically, the surgical approach is dorsal for an irreducible first MTP joint if the soft tissues allow [10,14,30].

Dislocations that involve disruption of the plantar structures can manifest themselves in many ways. Often, these dislocations are able to be reduced. Disruption can be seen as complete disruption of the plate from the proximal phalanx, longitudinal split, or some combination that involves a fracture of one of the sesamoids. Typically, repair of this injury is done surgically through a medial approach to the joint; one can access the dorsal and plantar aspects of the joint. The medial and plantar hallucal nerves should be watched for and avoided if possible. The plantar plate can be reapproximated to the proximal phalanx with suture through drill holes, and the intersesamoid ligament can be repaired with sutures. The sesamoids should be assessed for fracture.

Late sequelae

Late sequelae of turf toe injuries can occur after conservative treatment and, less commonly, after surgical treatment. Coker and colleagues [34] reported on nine athletes who sustained a hyperextension injury. The most common late sequelae were joint stiffness and pain with athletic activity. Clanton and colleagues [28] studied 20 patients who had turf toe injuries with a 5-year follow-up period, and noted persistent symptoms in 50% of cases. The same complication applies to sand toe injuries. Frey and colleagues [28] noted that after 6 months of rehabilitation, the most common problem was a loss of dorsiflexion (25% to 50%) with residual pain. Other late sequelae include a cock-up toe deformity, hallux rigidis, arthrofibrosis, loose bodies, traumatic bunion, and loss of push-off strength.

Sesamoid fractures

Anatomy

The sesamoids are an important part of the capsuloligamentous structure of the first MTP joint. They function within the joint complex as shock absorbers and fulcrums in supporting the weight-bearing portion of the first toe. Their

position on either side of the flexor hallucis longus forms a bony tunnel to protect the tendon (see Fig. 2) [35].

During the formation of the sesamoid, more than one ossification center
may be present, which may or may not unite. Multiple ossification centers give
rise to a partite sesamoid. The incidence of a partite medial sesamoid (tibial) is
roughly ten times that of a partite fibular sesamoid, with a prevalence of 5% to
30% in the general population. A partite sesamoid is seen bilaterally in 25% to
85% of patients with a documented partite sesamoid [36,37].

Diagnosis

A wide spectrum of injuries involves the sesamoids. These can include sesa-
moiditis, stress fractures, and acute fractures [35]. The mechanism of injury varies with the diagnosis. Direct blows, such as a fall from a height or a simple
landing from a jump (eg, in ballet), can cause acute fractures. Acute fractures also
can occur with axial loading seen with joint dislocations. Repetitive loading
from improper running usually gives rise to the more insidious stress fracture.
With repetitive loading, the fracture type typically is transverse in nature, whereas
the direct load–type injuries often are more comminuted and stellate.

Most often, pain is the patient's primary complaint. This pain is located directly under the first metatarsal head and is localized to the involved sesamoid.
Active or passive dorsiflexion of the first MTP joint can exacerbate the pain
because this puts stress on the osseous complex. The presence of a soft tissue
callus denotes a chronic process of the involved area.

AP, lateral, and sesamoid (tangential) views of the forefoot can be used for
diagnosis. The contralateral foot also must be visualized to compare the two
joints. This is most important if a partite sesamoid is being evaluated; however,
if the uninvolved foot does not have a partite sesamoid this does not confirm
the presence of a fracture [38].

Close inspection of the sesamoid in question is the best way to distinguish
between a partite sesamoid and an acute fracture. A partite sesamoid has smooth
sclerotic edges and the sum of its parts makes it larger than a normal sesamoid
(Fig. 6). Conversely, a fracture has a rough margin and is irregular (Fig. 7A). The
sum of the fragments should equal a normal sesamoid size. Also, fracture callus
can be seen on follow-up visits.

Injuries also can happen with a partite sesamoid. The synchondrosis of the
partite sesamoid may be stressed or may rupture. Stress views of the first MTP
joint in dorsiflexion can help to delineate this. Significant diastasis indicates at
least partial disruption of the plantar plate and may denotes plantar plate instability [31,39].

Treatment

The accepted treatment of any type of stable injury to the sesamoid alone
is conservative. Rest, ice, and elevation also can help. Immobilization may be

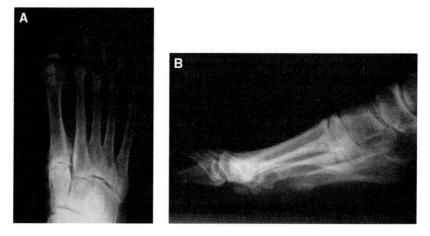

Fig. 6. AP (*A*) and lateral (*B*) radiographs of a bipartite sesamoid. Notice that the size of the two fragments together is much larger than a single sesamoid, and the edges are sclerotic and rounded.

needed to decrease the inflammation to the area. This can be done with a cast similar to that used for the management of turf toe. Often, a cast with a toe spica placed into slight plantarflexion so as to relax the plantar structures is useful. A midfoot ridge also can be helpful in removing excessive force onto the fore-foot. This altered weight bearing in a cast should be used for 4 to 6 weeks. As symptoms regress, the patient can advance his/her activity level. This might be

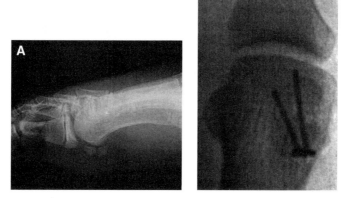

Fig. 7. (*A*) A sesamoid fracture in the lateral plane. Notice the ragged edges of the fracture. Also the sum of the fragments is equivalent to one sesamoid. (*B*) A sesamoid that has undergone open re-duction and internal fixation with a mini subchondral screw placed parallel to the metatarsosesamoid joint surface.

from a short leg cast into a stiff soled shoe. Complete relief of symptoms can take up to 6 months [40–42].

With prolonged symptoms and failed conservative therapy, excision of the involved sesamoid or bone grafting of the nonunited defect should be considered. Whenever possible, excision of only the distal pole of the fractured or diastased sesamoid has been the treatment of choice. This leaves a portion of the sesamoid for weight bearing. If symptoms persist, complete excision is performed, but it is not without complications. If the articular surface of the sesamoid is intact, and the cartilage is healthy, an attempt at open reduction with internal fixation—and possible bone grafting of the defect—should be undertaken (Fig. 7B) [43].

Typically, the medial sesamoid is approached through a medial incision. The joint is inspected for cartilage damage and congruity. For grafting the medial (tibial) sesamoid, the sesamoid should be approached just plantar to the insertion of the abductor hallucis tendon. Only the medial wall should be exposed. Minimal dissection should be done to preserve the blood supply to the sesamoid. A drill is used to disrupt the cortex and the void is filled with cancellous graft. A circumferential cerclage stitch of nonabsorbable suture should be placed around the sesamoid parallel to the joint surface and in the substance of the plantar plate. If the sesamoid is to be excised, it should be shelled out of the plantar plate carefully, and the void should be closed with suture. The short flexor brevis should be reconstructed and reinforced, if needed, to prevent deformity.

The lateral (fibular) sesamoid is much more difficult to access. Dorsal and plantar approaches have been described. Direct visualization of the joint surface and minimal disruption of blood supply occur with the dorsal approach. On approaching the lateral sesamoid, care should be taken to avoid the lateral plantar nerve just lateral to the sesamoid. Grafting should be done directly through this approach. If the sesamoid is going to be excised, the adductor tendon should be advanced into the distal aspect of the plantar plate for reinforcement.

At times, both sesamoids are involved; however, every effort should be made not to excise both sesamoids. With the excision of both sesamoids, the plantar complex loses a significant amount of function and mechanical advantage.

Postoperatively, care should mimic that of nonoperative care. The remaining sesamoid should be off-loaded until the healing has occurred. This can be done in a short leg cast or walker boot.

Complications

Nonunion of these fractures or irritated partite sesamoids can lead to significant pain and alteration of life activities and goals. Chronic pain despite appropriate treatment also is a problem. Both sesamoids can be removed; however, this can lead to significant problems. The imbalanced plantar mechanism can lead to hallux varus or valgus deformities as well as a cock-up toe deformity. These problems are best kept to a minimum by careful surgical skills and the proper use of orthotics.

Phalanx fractures

Anatomy

Like the first metatarsal, the first proximal phalanx is anatomically different from the lesser phalanges. The base of the first proximal phalanx is the attachment site of numerous tendons that include two short flexor tendon insertions, the adductor, the abductor, and the short extensor. The most powerful of these tendons is the short flexor tendons. These tendons work eccentrically to accept weight on the toe during mid and late stance [6].

Diagnosis

Phalangeal fractures are the most common fractures in the forefoot [10]. Mechanisms that are responsible for most of these fractures vary. A direct blow, such as a crush from a heavy object, usually causes a transverse or comminuted-type fracture. In the first ray, this injury is common among laborers. The short flexor tendons can cause a flexion deformity and lead to subsequent malunion and abnormal force distribution across the great toe [6]. An avulsion injury can occur on the proximal phalanx. Usually, this involves the plantarlateral corner of the proximal phalanx and is a significant fragment (20% of the joint surface) [6]. Often this piece is attached to the short flexor–adductor complex. This type of injury is common among athletes, such as gymnasts. A stubbing injury is the result of an axial load with a secondary varus or valgus stress that results in a spiral or oblique fracture pattern [10,44]. The stubbing mechanism is most likely to produce a clinical deformity [10].

Pain, ecchymosis, swelling, and difficulty walking barefoot are the usual presenting signs. Radiographic examination is needed to help differentiate between a sprain, dislocation, and fracture.

Fracture treatment

Treatment is conservative for most phalangeal fractures. Often, a stiff-soled shoe or immobilization is sufficient. All nondisplaced fractures, even intra-articular ones, can be managed like this initially. Some surgeons even advocate taping, although this seems to be more applicable to the lesser phalanges than to those of the first ray. The fractures that extend into the joint, especially the first MTP joint or the interphalangeal joint, should be opened and reduced properly. The first ray experiences at least twice as much weight as does any other ray.

Often, the surgical approach is dorsal and stays away from the plantar aspect of the great toe. For the intra-articular fractures that need to be reduced or the proximal phalangeal shaft that is malaligned, a direct approach often is indicated. Mini-screws, plates, or crossing k-wires may be used for fixation depending on the fracture pattern. For the plantarlateral fragment of the proximal phalanx, a dorsolateral incision is made to visualize the structures adequately to obtain a perfect reduction. A tension band construct can be used to augment the fixation and add compression [6].

Postoperatively, the hardware can be removed at roughly 4 weeks for k-wires and 8 to 12 weeks for screws and more definitive hardware. If a malunion occurs or arthrosis develops, conservative management is the rule with orthotics and anti-inflammatory drugs. If this is unsuccessful, fusion may become an option.

Summary

The spectrum of first ray injuries is broad and ranges from high-energy fractures to mild sprains and strains of the MTP joint. The impact on work and athletics is immense; therefore, these injuries should not be taken lightly.

Fractures of the first ray are not the same as those of the lesser toes. The first ray plays a significant role in maintaining normal function of the foot, and therefore, is not as forgiving as the lesser toes. Treatment must be slightly more aggressive than with the other rays. Fractures must be reduced and their anatomic relationships must be maintained. Hyperextension (turf toe) and hyper-flexion injuries (sand toe) also can be debilitating and lead to significant impairment. Most of these injuries, however, respond to rest, ice, taping, and elevation. Finally, all dislocations should undergo a trial reduction. The physician should be aware that although a type I dislocation looks benign, open reduction probably will be required.

References

[1] Sammarco GJ. Biomechanics of the foot. In: Frankel VH, Nordin M, editors. Basic biomechanics of the skeletal system. Philadelphia: Lea & Febiger; 1980. p. 193–220.

[2] Saraiya M. First metatarsal fractures. Clin Podiatr Med Surg 1995;12(4):749–58.

[3] Bohay DR, Johnson KD, Manoli II A. The traumatic bunion. Foot Ankle Int 1996;17(7):383–7.

[4] Goossens M, DeStoop N. Lisfranc fracture-dislocations: a review of 20 cases. Clin Orthop Rel Res 1983;176:154–62.

[5] Sangeorzan BJ, Hansen Jr ST. Early and late foot reconstruction. Clin Orthop Rel Res 1989; 243:86–91.

[6] Hansen Jr ST. Functional reconstruction of the foot and ankle. Philadelphia: Lippincott Williams & Wilkins; 2000.

[7] Johnson VS. Treatment of fractures of the forefoot in industry. In: Bateman J, editor. Foot science. Philadelphia: WB Saunders; 1976.

[8] Giannestras NJ, Sammarco GJ. Fractures and dislocations of the foot. In: Rockwood CA, Green DP, editors. Fractures. Philadelphia: JB Lippincott; 2001. p. 1400.

[9] Garcia A, Parks JC. Fractures of the foot. In: Giannestra S, editor. Foot disorders, medical and surgical management. 2nd edition. Philadelphia: Lea & Febiger; 1973. p. 517–29.

[10] Early JS. Fractures and dislocations of the midfoot and forefoot. In: Bucholz R, Heckman J, editors. Fractures in adults. 5th edition. Philadelphia: WB Saunders; 2001. p. 2217–21.

[11] LaPorta G. Fracture of the first metatarsal. In: Scurran BL, editor. Foot and ankle trauma. New York: Churchill Livingstone; 1989. p. 323–45.

[12] Mann RA, Coughlin JM. Surgery of the foot and ankle. 6th edition. St. Louis, Missouri: Mosby Inc.; 1993.

[13] Bowers KD, Martin RB. Turf-toe: a shoe-surface related football injury. Med Sci Sports 1976; 8:81–3.

[14] Watson TS, Anderson RB, Davis WH. Periarticular injuries to the hallux metatarsophalangeal joint in athletes. Foot Ankle Clin 2000;5(3):687–713.

[15] Hetherington VJ, Carnett J, Patterson BA. Motion of the first metatarsophalangeal joint. J Foot Surg 1989;28:13–9.

[16] Stokes AF, Hutton WC, Scott JR. Forces under the hallux valgus foot before and after surgery. Clin Orthop Rel Res 1979;142:64–72.

[17] Nigg BM. Biomechanical aspects of running. Biomechanics of running shoes. Champaign (IL): Humana Kinetics; 1986. p. 1–25.

[18] Joseph J. Range of movement of the great toe in men. J Bone Joint Surg Br 1954;36:450–7.

[19] Bojsen-Miller F, Lamoreux L. Significance of free dorsiflexion of the toes in walking. Acta Orthop Scand 1979;50:471–9.

[20] Bowman MW. Athletic injuries of the great toe metatarsophalangeal joint. In: Anderson RB, Adelaar MD, editors. Disorders of the great toe, monograph series. Rosemont (IL): American Academy of Orthopaedic Surgeons; 1997. p. 1–22.

[21] Rodeo SA, O'Brien S, Warren RF. Turf-toe: an analysis of metatarsophalangeal joint sprains in professional football players. Am J Sports Med 1990;18:280–5.

[22] Nigg BM, Segesser B. The influence of playing surfaces on the load on the locomotor system and on football and tennis injuries. Sports Med 1988;5:375–85.

[23] Clanton TO. Athletic injuries to the soft tissues of the foot and ankle. In: Coughlin MJ, Mann RA, editors. 7th edition. Surgery of the foot and ankle, vol. 2. St. Louis (MO): Mosby; 1999. p. 1175–88.

[24] Clanton TO, Butler JE, Eggert A. Injuries to the metarsophalangeal joint in athletes. Foot Ankle 1986;7:162–76.

[25] Douglas DI, Davidson DM, Robinson JE. Rupture of the medial collateral ligament of the first metatarsophalangeal joint in a professional soccer player. J Foot Ankle Surg 1997;36:388–90.

[26] Mullis OL, Miller WE. A disabling sports injury of the great toe. Foot Ankle 1980;1:22–5.

[27] Clanton TO, Ford JJ. Turf toe injury. Clin Sports Med 1994;13(4):731–41.

[28] Frey C, Andersen GD, Feder KS. Plantarflexion injury to the metatarsophalangeal joint ("sand toe"). Foot Ankle 1996;17:576–81.

[29] Sammarco GJ. How I manage turf toe. Phys Sportsmed 1988;16:113–8.

[30] Brunet J. Pathomechanics of complex dislocations of the first metatarsophalangeal joint. Clin Orthop Rel Res 1996;332:1126–31.

[31] Hall R, Saxby T, Vandemark R. A new type of dislocation of the first metatarsophalangeal joint: a case report. Foot Ankle Int 1992;13(9):540–5.

[32] Jahss M. Traumatic dislocation of the first metatarsophalangeal joint. Foot Ankle Int 1980;1(1): 15–21.

[33] Nabarro M, Powell J. Dorsal dislocation of the metatarsophalangeal joint of the great toe. Foot Ankle Int 1995;16(2):75–8.

[34] Coker TI, Arnold JA, Weber DL. Traumatic lesions of the metatarsophalangeal joint of the great toe in athletes. Am J Sports Med 1978;6:326–34.

[35] Beaman D, Saltzman C. Disorders of the hallucal sesamoids. In: Anderson RB, Adelaar MD, editors. Disorders of the great toe, monograph series. Rosemont (IL): American Academy of Orthopedic Surgeons; 1997. p. 33–41.

[36] Chisin D, Peyser A, Milgram C. Bone scintigraphy in the assessment of hallucal sesamoids. Foot Ankle Int 1995;16:291–4.

[37] Jahss M. The sesamoids of the hallux. Clin Orthop Rel Res 1981;157:88–97.

[38] Prieskorn D, Graves S, Smith R. Morphometric analysis of plantar plate apparatus. Foot Ankle Int 1993;14(4):204–7.

[39] Rodeo S, Warren N, O'Brien S. Diastasis of bipartite sesamoids of the first metatarsophalangeal joint. Foot Ankle Int 1992;13:277–81.

[40] McBryde A, Anderson R. Sesamoid foot problems in the athlete. Clin Sports Med 1988;7: 51–60.

[41] Van Hall M, Keene J, Lange T. Stress fractures of the great toe sesamoids. Am J Sports Med 1982;10:122–8.

[42] Weiss J. Fracture of the medial sesamoid bone of the great toe: controversies in therapy. Orthopedics 1991;14:1003–7.

[43] Anderson R, McBryde A. Autogenous bone grafting of hallux sesamoid nonunions. Foot Ankle Int 1997;18(5):293–6.

[44] Hansen ST. Foot injuries. In: Browner BD, Jupiter JB, editors. Skeletal trauma, vol. 2. Philadelphia: WB Saunders; 1998. p. 2405–38.

ELSEVIER
SAUNDERS

Foot Ankle Clin N Am
11 (2006) 165–182

FOOT AND
ANKLE CLINICS

Foot and Ankle Reconstruction After Blast Injuries

Francis X. McGuigan, MD[a,b],*, Jonathan A. Forsberg, MD[a,b],
Romney C. Andersen, MD[a,b]

[a]Department of Orthopaedic Surgery, National Naval Medical Center, 8901 Wisconsin Avenue,
Bethesda, MD 20889, USA
[b]Uniformed Services University of the Health Sciences, 4301 Jones Bridge Road,
Bethesda, MD 20814, USA

The war on terrorism is producing the largest number of gravely injured soldiers and Marines since the end of the Viet Nam conflict. Through September 2005, more than 17,000 casualties resulted from combat operations in Iraq and Afghanistan. A total of 7200 servicemen and women were injured severely enough that they could not return to combat action within 72 hours [1]. Over 70% of these casualties involved extremity trauma and comminuted open fractures with severely compromised soft tissue envelopes. Most of these penetrating injuries were not caused by bullets but rather by exploding ordnance, primarily improvised explosive devices (IEDs).

Extremity wounds have become the most common type of injury inflicted on American and Allied troops [2–9]. Two recent changes in armed conflict are responsible for this phenomenon. The first change is in the type of body armor worn by service members. Kevlar body armor has evolved over the past 40 years, providing significant protection to a combatant's head, chest, abdomen, and groin. The addition of ceramic plating makes body armor almost impenetrable to even high velocity ammunition rounds. Body armor adequately protects the brain and vital organs from penetrating injury but leaves the extremities exposed;

No author has any relationship with or any financial interest in any product discussed within this article. No funding was received from any source toward the preparation of this article. The opinions expressed herein are those of the authors and are not necessarily representative of those of the National Naval Medical Center, the Department of Defense, or the United States Army or Navy.

* Corresponding author. Department of Orthopaedic Surgery, National Naval Medical Center, 8901 Wisconsin Avenue, Bethesda, MD 20889.

E-mail address: fxmcguigan@bethesda.med.navy.mil (F.X. McGuigan).

1083-7515/06/$ – see front matter. Published by Elsevier Inc.
doi:10.1016/j.fcl.2005.10.002

therefore, advances in body armor have produced a distinct injury pattern. Patient survivability improves at the cost of unprecedented numbers of mangled extremities. The second change in armed conflict that has increased the incidence of extremity injuries is the enemy's choice of weaponry. Explosive devices are increasingly popular owing to their low cost, devastating effects, and ease of manufacture. In Iraq, IEDs are the weapon of choice of the insurgency because they are detonated remotely with little or no risk to the insurgents while inflicting devastating injuries on the intended victims. Casualties that result from explosive ordinance are associated with a higher proportion of orthopedic injuries than seen in prior conflicts fought primarily with conventional firearms [5–8,10–12]. Conventional firearms target the chest and abdomen, whereas fragmentary projectiles from a blast target all body areas, including the extremities [12,13].

Historical perspective on limb salvage in wartime

Each major armed conflict results in advances in the orthopedic care of combat casualties and in techniques of lower extremity limb salvage. In 1861, amputation was recommended for open fractures, major nerve or blood vessel damage, extensive soft tissue injury, or arthrotomy [14]. During the First World War, amputation rates after blast injury to the extremities approached 75% [15]. The overall rate of limb salvage during the past 80 years has improved with better operative techniques, improvements in anesthesia, the discovery of antibiotics, and the use blood transfusions [16,17]. The discovery of the anticoagulant sodium citrate made banked blood possible for the first time at the end of the First World War, saving thousand of lives. The introduction of external fixation by Anderson and Hoffman advanced the ability to treat the soft tissue component of open fractures [18,19]. The Second World War witnessed the first large-scale use of antibiotics in the treatment of battle injuries, reducing the amputation rate to 50% [20].

The Korean conflict saw the advent of helicopter evacuation to forward surgical units, decreasing the time from injury to operative intervention and reducing mortality from exsanguination. The amputation rate during the Korean Conflict decreased to 18% of all extremity injuries, partly attributable to the new technique of vascular repair [21,22]. In Viet Nam, military surgeons routinely performed vascular repairs and reconstructions on extremity wounds, making limb salvage a viable option for even severely injured extremities [10,23,24]. The lower extremity amputation rate has decreased to 14% in the most recent conflicts (Box 1) [9,10,25,26].

It is unknown whether the limb salvage rate can be improved further in the current conflict because of the severity of the injuries and the improvements in prosthetics. Extremity injuries in the global war on terrorism are more severe than injuries in previous armed conflicts owing to the high number of blast injuries. Improvements made in prosthetic technology have resulted in amputees achieving a higher level of function, making amputation a more viable

---

Box 1. Lower extremity amputation rates in recent armed conflicts (*low numbers of injured extremities)

Somalia, 14%*
Desert Storm, 14%
Grenada, 19%*
Viet Nam, 12.7%
Korea, 17.9%
WWII, 50%

---

alternative. The percentage of amputations performed in the current conflict, therefore, may not necessarily reflect recent technical advances in limb salvage surgery [9].

Blast injury pathomechanics

Blast injuries are associated with unique soft tissue challenges, increasing the complexity of skeletal injury when compared with similar fracture patterns treated in a civilian trauma setting. These high-energy penetrating injuries result in a massive zone of injury, the presence of foreign bodies, and gross contamination with multiply resistant environmental bacteria. Blast-related projectiles travel at low velocities (<600 m/s), but the fragments are large, and their increased mass imparts greater kinetic force than low velocity gun shot wounds ($Ke = \frac{1}{2}mv^2$). These fragments are irregular in shape, causing more tissue tearing and crushing. The fragments tumble, adding to the soft tissue injury. The blast propels scrapnel, environmental debris, pieces of clothing, and shoe wear into the wound sites, imparting a massive bacterial load.

Multidisciplinary effort

The treatment of blast-induced extremity trauma is truly a multidisciplinary effort requiring the formation of a large comprehensive team (Box 2). Each member of this team contributes valuable expertise in the care of the injured service member. The patient is also an integral member of the team and must be educated and counseled appropriately to make the ultimate decision regarding limb salvage or amputation.

Stages of treatment

The stages of treatment of lower extremity blast injuries are listed in Box 3.

Box 2. Comprehensive multidisciplinary approach

The patient
Anesthesia and the pain service
Critical care medicine
Infectious disease
Clinical nutrition
Orthopedic surgery
Physical and occupational therapy
Plastic surgery
Prosthetics
Military liaison
Mental health
Physical medicine and rehabilitation
Pastoral care
Radiology
Social work
Trauma/general surgery
Vascular surgery

Initial assessment and clinical examination

Following the medical evacuation from overseas treatment facilities the initial evaluation of casualties in the receiving medical center is performed by the trauma/general surgery team. The trauma team directs the evaluation process, prioritizing care and consulting the appropriate surgical and medical services. The orthopedic evaluation includes a complete secondary survey. A "hand-over-hand" examination is performed with particular attention to joints and extremities that have not been addressed surgically to identify frequently missed injuries such as joint dislocations, closed fractures, and compartment syndrome. Compartment syndromes of the foot are one of the most frequently overlooked injuries and

Box 3. Stages of treatment

Initial assessment and clinical examination
Consider amputation
Serial debridements
Eradication of infection
Soft tissue coverage
Fracture fixation
Treatment of bone defects
Secondary reconstructive procedures

conditions. In cases of significant hindfoot trauma, a complete decompression of the foot compartments requires a tarsal tunnel release [27]. Extremity splints and dressings are removed to determine the status of all wounds and the need for urgent debridement. A comprehensive orthopedic examination may also uncover decubitus ulcers or small blast wound infections that may have developed in transit. The vascular status of all extremities is determined. For patients who are awake and compliant, a careful neurologic examination is performed. It is vital that the injured service member be reassessed throughout the initial days of the hospitalization to uncover additional injuries and to note changes in the neurologic and vascular status. A complete history is also vital because even though most active duty service members are young and free of significant co-morbidities, this may not be true for members of reserve forces. A large per-centage of the fighting force uses tobacco products. The negative role tobacco products have in healing is discussed with the service member. Cessation of tobacco use is an important first step in limb salvage.

Imaging studies are a key part of the orthopedic examination of blast injuries. Standard radiographs delineate not only the character of the fracture but also the presence of metallic fragments. Debris travels along fascial planes and can lodge in soft tissues far from the entry wound. Contaminated debris requiring removal may be seen as intermediate density lesions. CT scans aid the assessment of intra-articular fractures. Metal suppression techniques are required to decrease scatter. Three-dimensional reconstruction images can guide orthopedic procedures in complex cases but are not always necessary. MRI has little value in the acute setting of blast injuries. Metallic artifact limits MRI use within the first 6 weeks following the injury until metallic fragments become stabilized by scar formation. After the initial phases of treatment are complete, MRI is valuable in determining the extent of soft tissue and bone infections. Angiograms are used to determine the vascular status of a limb, especially as a prelude to free flap procedures.

Consider amputation

Despite advances in limb salvage surgery, there are instances when amputation is a better option for a potentially salvageable limb because the limb saved will be severely limited functionally. Preservation of the limb is not the only benchmark for success in the treatment of these injuries, because the functional result of a salvaged limb may not meet patient expectations. Prosthetic improvements using composite materials, energy storing designs, and microprocessors allow many unilateral lower extremity amputees to achieve greater functional recovery than their limb salvage counterparts. In patients with severely injured limbs, early consultation with the patient regarding realistic expectations is paramount. Probable outcomes of limb salvage and amputation should be discussed frankly to help the patient decide on the appropriate treatment plan. Successful counseling may prevent prolonged disability resulting from an overly optimistic salvage. Interviews with amputees and service members who have undergone limb salvage are offered to the service member and his or her family to aid in decision making.

Most of the trauma literature on lower extremity amputation comes from the treatment of open tibia fractures. Absolute indications for primary limb amputation include systemic sepsis or irreparable vascular injury. Lange and coworkers [28] and Hansen [29] consider the loss of arterial inflow for greater than 6 hours and disruption of the posterior tibial nerve to be an indication for early amputation. In patients with grade IIIC tibia fractures, immediate amputation is also warranted if any two of the following characteristics are present: serious associated polytrauma, severe ipsilateral foot trauma, a protracted course to obtain soft tissue coverage, or the need for tibial bone reconstruction. Open tibial fractures associated with a proximal vascular injury and repair are difficult to treat and portend a bad prognosis. The amputation rate for these injuries is between 36% and 78% [30,31]. Injury factors that influence the decision to amputate in cases of open tibial fractures include the fracture pattern, the presence of an open foot fracture, bone loss, muscle injury, vein injury, arterial injury, and the absence of plantar sensation [32].

Although complete loss of plantar sensation is considered an indication for amputation, this indication must be used cautiously in the treatment of blast injuries. Many patients present with a reversible loss in plantar sensation, a neuropraxia, or an axonotmesis owing to the blast or surgical debridement that resolves in a period of months. Others may not possess normal plantar sensation but may have sufficient protective sensation over a portion of the foot to permit a good functional outcome. Many nerve injuries, especially of the tibial nerve at the ankle, occur in areas that may be amenable to nerve grafting.

Impaired foot and ankle function is a relative indication for below knee or Syme amputation. Ipsilateral loss of the ankle and subtalar joint, when accompanied by discontinuity of the forefoot, is a difficult reconstructive challenge. Loss of multiple muscle compartments in the leg through devitalization, dennervation, or transection of muscles and tendons is another injury pattern that results in suboptimal functioning of the residual limb through loss of active and passive motion and progressive ankle deformity owing to tendon imbalance. The status of the contralateral limb is a significant variable in determining whether limb salvage should be attempted. If removal of the limb results in bilateral amputations, especially above the knee, limb salvage may be preferable because expenditure for ambulation is considerable.

Amputation is not a panacea. Poor outcomes after amputation can occur when wound infection and dehiscence result in shorter limb length, loss of the gastrosoleus muscle flap, and poor skin envelopes. Formation of heterotopic ossification and failure of a myodesis may require revision surgery. Neuroma formation or a complex regional pain syndrome may limit the amputee's physical goals and prevent prosthetic fitting.

Occasionally, amputees are able to return to active duty. Service members must achieve and maintain a high level of physical function to return to the field. An Ertl amputation may be an advantage in this regard (Fig. 1). The osteo-

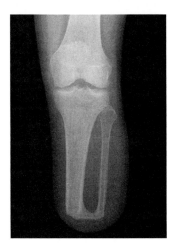

Fig. 1. Ertl amputation.

myoplasty uses an osteoperiosteal bridge to create a distal synostosis between the residual tibia and fibula, theoretically producing a stump with better function [33–35].

A multicenter study is underway to categorize the war injuries of all service members and to determine the long-term outcome of their treatment. In the future, it may be clear what combination of bone and soft tissue injuries does best with amputation and what combination does well with limb salvage.

Serial debridements

The debridement technique is the same as that employed in many civilian trauma settings, but tissue removal is more aggressive. Traumatic wounds are extended to provide adequate visualization. All nonmetallic foreign body debris is removed. Devitalized muscle (based on color, contractility, consistency, and bleeding), fascia, and fat are excised. Charred or devitalized bone (free bone without muscle attachment) is removed. Deep tissue and exudates are sent for culture following debridement. High-pressure irrigation with 3 to 6 L of normal saline is followed by 3 L of bacitracin-laden normal saline or a castile soap solution [36]. Pulsatile lavage may devitalize bone and traumatize tissues when used in repetitive debridements. Neurovascular structures are covered following debridement and irrigation to prevent nerve irritation and vessel desiccation. Antibiotic-impregnated polymethyl methacrylate (PMMA) beads or spacers are placed within the wound. Deep layers are closed using monofilament absorbable sutures. Skin is closed using nylon.

Vacuum assisted closure (VAC) dressings provide negative pressure wound therapy and are useful in treating open injuries by extracting serum and reducing bacterial counts. A carbon-impregnated sponge is placed over the wound and secured with staples under an occlusive membrane. Suction via a catheter exerts a negative pressure of 120 mm Hg. The VAC is used for dressing open wounds, split-thickness skin grafts, and the incision lines around muscle flaps. In addition to avoiding bulky exudate-soaked dressings, negative pressure wound therapy is thought to promote granulation tissue formation and to draw wounds closed uniformly.

Eradication of infection

All blast fractures are considered infected. As many as 75% of blast injuries are culture positive, often with exotic bacteria. The collective bacteriologic bioburden may range from simple contamination to fulminate infection that significantly impedes wound healing [37]. Routine Gram stains and surface cultures are not necessarily representative of the predominant organism causing the deep infection [38–40] or of the bacterial load [41,42]. Differentiating between colonization and clinically significant infection is based on clinical response and history. Most blast injuries result in polymicrobial infections. The constellation of organisms observed is similar to that seen in grossly contaminated wounds in civilian trauma but also includes exotic environmental pathogens such as *Acinetobacter baumannii* [43]. *Acinetobacter* is a gram-negative bacillus commonly found in soil. It was the most common bacteria found in Viet Nam combat injuries and is the most prevalent in the current conflict. *Acinetobacter* is resistant to many antibiotics, including imipenem (18%), amikacin (52%), ampicillin sodium/sulbactam sodium (65%), cefepime (78%), and ciprofloxacin (80%). Four percent of infections are resistant to all antibiotics [43]. Universal contact precautions must be taken when *Acinetobacter* is identified as a pathogen [44].

Antibiotic impregnated beads and spacers

The use of antibiotic-impregnated beads or spacers in conjunction with parenteral antibiotics increases the chance of infection eradication. Antibiotic-impregnated PMMA beads deliver high local tissue concentrations of antibiotics without the systemic toxicity associated with intravenous application [45–50]. Recent foot and ankle publications describe the use of PMMA beads to treat soft tissue infections and osteomyelitis [51–53]. Based on the results of initial cultures, vancomycin, 1 g, tobramycin, 2.4 g, or iminipenem alone or in combination are used per packet of Palacos R (Zimmer, Warsaw, Indiana) polymer to form the beads or spacers. In several studies, Palacos R demonstrated an increased elution of antibiotics when compared with other formulations of PMMA [54–57]. In the foot and ankle, antibiotic-impregnated PMMA spacer blocks are preferable to beads to fill the osseous void created by the projectile and to hold the soft tissues at normal tension. The use of antibiotic-impregnated PMMA is a mainstay treatment of wartime open lower extremity trauma.

Other biodegradeable antibiotic carrying agents in development are hydroxyapatite, polylactic acid, poly (DL-lactide) coglycolide, glass-polymer composites, and sponge collagen. A higher concentration of antibiotics is delivered for a greater length of time than when using PMMA [58–61]. Potentially, a single stage reconstruction may be performed using these devices, but the severity of most blast injuries makes this unlikely. The current generation of biodegradable implants also lacks the stability and moldability desirable for use as an antibiotic-impregnated spacer block.

Specialized dressings

Aquacel Ag (Convatec/Bristol-Myers Squibb, Princeton, New Jersey) is a silver nitrate–impregnated dressing that is particularly beneficial for use in extensive full-thickness wounds that produce large quantities of exudate. This dressing promotes fluid absorption and locks bacteria within "gelled fibers" away from the wound bed. The silver possesses antimicrobial activity and acts against *Pseudomonas aeruginosa*, methicillin-resistant *Staphylococcus aureus*, and vancomycin-resistant enterococcus. In several instances, use of the Aquacel Ag dressing appeared to alter favorably the course of wounds that did not respond to intravenous antibiotics, antibiotic beads, and serial debridement.

Infection monitoring

Determination of when it is safe to perform closure of an infected blast wound is subjective and inexact. Deep cultures are taken at the end of every surgical debridement. Negative culture results, however, are equivocal in light of intravenous antibiotic administration. White blood cell counts, sedimentation rates, and C-reactive protein levels are unfortunately dependent on systemic as well as local factors. Matched bone scintigraphy and indium scans have significant false-negative and positive rates in determining the presence of osteomyelitis. MRI can be useful in determining early osteomyelitis, but in the presence of shrapnel, its use must be delayed for 6 weeks following injury. Determination of wound closure is dependent on the subjective clinical experience of the team rather than objective test criteria.

Avoiding secondary soft tissue injuries

Secondary soft tissue injuries and complications must be avoided. Heel pressure ulcers may occur during evacuation. Most service members with open lower extremity fractures undergo medical evacuation from the area of combat operations with a unilateral external fixator in place. The heel is in a dependent position and takes the weight of the entire extremity during hospitalization and multiple transfers. "Kick stands" added to external fixation keep the skin clear of the bed, eliminating the risk of heel ulcers. Sacral decubitus is a less prevalent complication.

Many extremities are tenuously close to being avascular; therefore, care must be taken when applying lower extremity dressings and elevating limbs. Plaster splints may cause vascular insufficiency as cotton webbing soaked with blood dries, causing constriction. VAC dressings placed circumferentially are also a potential risk. Some limbs have been observed to develop an "elevation induced" loss of arterial pulse. The combination of a traumatized extended limb, hypotension, external fixation, and excessive elevation produces a loss of arterial pulse. Extremity elevation after injury should be to the level of the heart only.

Soft tissue coverage

Fasciocutaneous flaps, rotational muscle flaps, or free flaps may be required to achieve infection eradication and bone union. Local infection control by serial debridements to a level of 10^5 organisms per gram of tissue before the flap procedure is noted to correlate with success [62]. Fasciocutaneous flaps (dorsalis pedis, reverse sural, free anterolateral thigh, medial plantar, and medial calcaneal) can provide skin coverage in areas of minimal bone destruction and a sufficient muscle bed. The skin from adjacent digits that are not salvageable can serve as vascularized full-thickness grafts. Although the plastic surgery consultant makes the ultimate choice of flap procedure, fasciocutaneous coverage may not eradicate bone infection and heal fractures in areas devoid of an appropriate muscle bed. Muscle flaps decrease bacterial counts, increase blood supply, and promote bone healing and are preferable to fasciocutaneous flaps from the orthopedic viewpoint.

Muscle rotation flaps of the gastrocnemius, soleus, peroneal muscles, and extensor digitorum brevis provide coverage for open fractures of the leg and foot. In the distal aspect of the lower extremity, free muscle flaps are required using a free rectus abdominus graft, although the gracilis and partial serratus anterior flaps are also useful. In a civilian trauma setting, flap coverage procedures are usually accomplished within 72 hours [63]. In military blast injuries, flap coverage is performed later because of medical evacuation and to allow for serial debridement of infected and devitalized tissue. Unfortunately, late flap coverage carries higher rates of bone nonunion, osteomyelitis, and flap failure [63,64].

Fracture fixation

In some instances, a fracture is minor or stable enough to avoid the use of internal fixation; however, most fractures require fixation to achieve the recognized objectives of fracture treatment. Standard AO techniques in the treatment of open fractures may increase soft tissue injury and risk ongoing infection owing to exposed hardware. Minimally invasive techniques still possess these disadvantages. Intramedullary fixation for most blast-induced open fractures is not indicated. The ideal fixation method for the treatment of these open fractures would avoid internal fixation; minimize soft tissue trauma; restore articular surfaces; maintain limb alignment, rotation, and length; permit ongoing soft tissue restoration; permit early weight bearing; and preserve joint mobility. A combined approach with limited internal fixation for restoration of joint surfaces and external fixation for limb stabilization seems best to achieve these goals.

The use of monolateral external fixators for high-energy blast injuries in mobile surgical units and fixed forward hospitals has proven efficacy [65–70]. Monolateral external fixators span soft tissue injuries and stabilize fractures while allowing soft tissue access for further surgical intervention and wound care. External fixators minimize further soft tissue injury by avoiding the periosteal stripping associated with internal fixation and preserving the intramedulary blood supply compromised by rods. External fixators provide necessary stability while minimizing the risk of infection and osteomyelitis associated with retained internal hardware.

Monolateral external fixators have significant drawbacks in the treatment of open lower extremity fractures. They are generally not rigid enough to permit early unrestricted weight bearing. Monolateral external fixation requires spanning constructs in the treatment of periarticular fractures. Monolateral constructs impose severe limitations in the correction of limb rotation, translation, angulation, and length. Monolateral fixator pins are also prone to loosening and infection during the prolonged treatment period required for healing blast-induced fractures.

Ring fixators overcome many of the limitations inherent in monolateral external fixators while still offering the advantages of bone stabilization and soft tissue access [71]. They allow immediate weight bearing and have more options for selecting pin site orientation, which is important in limbs with severely injured soft tissue envelopes. The frames can be constructed to allow motion of joints immediately adjacent to the fracture. The ability to shorten acutely a limb with a ring fixator may also obviate the need for rotation and free flap procedures. Ring fixators can be used for limb lengthening procedures to compensate for bone deficits and can address rotational and angular deformities.

Ring fixation for the treatment of periarticular fractures may require wire fixation for fracture stabilization. For metadiaphyseal and diaphyseal fractures, half pins offer advantages in strength and simplicity. Half pins increase patient tolerance of the frames. Conventional half pins may become loose or infected when used for extended periods. Hydroxyapatite coatings have prolonged the longevity of half pins [72]. In one study with a mean implantation time of 530 days, the rate of half pin loosening was 4% for coated pins and 80% for uncoated pins [73].

The Taylor Spatial Frame ring fixator (TSF) (Smith & Nephew, Memphis, Tennessee) possesses unique features that further increase the appeal of ring fixators as the definitive fixation of blast injuries below the knee. The basic TSF device consists of six obliquely oriented struts connected between two rings that can generate six axes of deformity corrections. The frame application is much faster and simpler than the standard Ilizarov technique. Postoperative corrections are achieved by the use of computer software resulting in anatomic restoration of limb alignment and joint orientation. SpatialCad (Orthocrat, Houston, Texas) software can be used to first digitalize radiographs and then define the parameters of the deformity. This information is uploaded to a TSF website (https://www.spatialframe.com) along with the details of the frame construct. A schedule for frame adjustment to correct the deformity is generated based on identified structures at risk or a set timetable for deformity correction. The TSF ring fixator allows treatment of soft tissue and bone defects not possible with other fixation methods (Figs. 2 to 4).

Conversion from a temporary monolateral fixator to a ring fixator should be considered when serial debridements are complete, infection is controlled, and

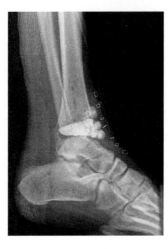

Fig. 2. Lateral ankle radiograph with PMMA spacers in place following open tibial plafond fracture with loss of extensor mechanism. Patient also sustained an ipsilateral open tibial plateau fracture and contralateral traumatic above knee amputation.

flaps are able to survive further surgical interventions. The timing of frame conversion averages depends on the clinical situation. It typically occurs 10 days following the initial injury or definitive flap procedure.

Treatment of bone defects

Bone defects below the knee are often large, multifocal, and associated with articular cartilage and soft tissue loss. Reconstruction is performed after infection eradication. Bone defects are treated by autografting, allografting, lengthening, or shortening. Staged reconstructions are time consuming and can be

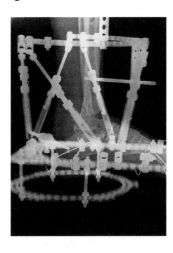

Fig. 3. Lateral ankle radiograph with TSF frame in place.

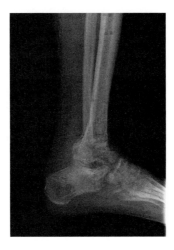

Fig. 4. Lateral ankle radiograph following frame removal.

frustrating, especially for young service members eager to return to duty or complete rehabilitation.

Diaphyseal and metadiaphyseal bone loss of 5 cm or more usually requires bone lengthening or transport procedures. In these situations, a corticotomy away from the area of injury is preferred. A double corticotomy will shorten the time of lengthening by half and decrease the time until frame removal. After the completion of the lengthening phase, it may be necessary to bone graft the docking site. The poor tissue envelopes and the prevalence of heterotopic ossification associated with blast injuries make these lengthenings technically challenging.

Diaphyseal and metadiaphyseal deficits less than 5 cm with a ring fixator in place can be treated with morselized autograft or cancellous allograft combined with recombinant bone morphogenetic protein. InFUSE (Medtronic, Minneapolis, Minnesota) is a recombinant human bone morphogenetic protein (rhBMP-2) with proven clinical success in the treatment of acute tibial fractures equal to that of autograft bone [74]. Bone deficits less than 2 cm may not require any measures to restore limb length.

Fractures of the ankle and foot with residual bone deficits require more specialized decision making than open tibial fractures. In rare instances, immediate attempts at primary fusion of the ankle, subtalar joint, or tarsal bones can be performed, providing that these procedures can be accomplished without bone graft or internal fixation. The articular surfaces are denuded, and the foot is held in place with a ring fixator to achieve compression and to allow weight bearing. Treatment of talus fractures with complete or partial loss of the body or head is further complicated by avascular necrosis. Fusion between the avascular talar fragment and the tibia or midfoot is extremely difficult. These fractures require staged reconstructions with delayed bone grafting and internal fixation. Bone deficits in the foot are treated with internal fixation and bone grafting following a period of soft tissue healing and graft maturation. The process is facilitated if an antibiotic spacer is used to fill the initial bone defect. The spacer is removed, the cavity is debrided of fibrous tissue, and the bone surfaces are burred to bleeding bone. The void is filled with cancellous autograft or allograft bone supplemented with recombinant bone morphogenetic protein. Internal fixation is then performed using standard fixation techniques or locking plates. Locking plates provide stable fixation in the foot despite severe bone deficiencies, particularly when limited surface area is available for fixation or the bone available for fixation is poor.

Secondary reconstructive procedures

Although it is useful to think of the initial phases of treatment and secondary reconstructive procedures as two distinct stages of treatment, they are a continuum. Success in the reconstructive phase depends on achieving the goals of the initial phases of treatment. Tendon transfers will not benefit the patient when infection is not cleared, wounds have not healed, and joints are constrained by fixation. There is a delicate balance between a too aggressive surgical approach for the degree of injury and a too timid approach that compromises reconstructive options and functional return.

Occupational therapy, physical therapy and adjuvant measures are vital to preserve reconstructive options before the definitive procedures. Loss of motion in the foot and ankle increases joint forces and alters kinematics of the hip and knee. Tendon imbalance, which leads to equinus or varus contracture, must be braced until tendon transfers are performed. Limb edema creates joint contractures and tenosynovial adhesions, particularly in the foot digits, which are often neglected in physical therapy. The use of compression stockings following soft tissue stabilization may minimize the edema that limits motion and creates stiffness. Heterotopic ossification and muscle fibrosis can also tether and restrict articulations. Instructing the injured service member and his or her family in joint mobilization exercises assists the efforts of physical and occupational therapy in restoring joint motion.

Secondary reconstructive procedures are tailored to the individual blast injury pattern. Late osteotomies or joint fusions are accomplished in standard fashion with due consideration to the increased risk of recurrent infection, the limitations of an impaired soft tissue envelope, and the problems inherent in significant bone loss. Most soft tissue procedures are similar to those performed in a civilian foot and ankle practice, such as claw toe releases, tendoachilles lengthenings/ augmentations, and split anterior tibialis tendon transfers. Some of the less common procedures for tendon imbalance include anterior transfer of the posterior tibial tendon and transfer of the peroneus longus to the calcaneus. An area of muscle fibrosis and tendon entrapment may be bypassed using Alloderm (Lifecell, Branchburg, New Jersey). Cartilage replacement procedures and total ankle arthroplasty are more controversial in the reconstruction of the severely traumatized limb and have not been attempted.

Pain and psychologic trauma

These injuries require expert pain management. The neurogenic pain associated with blast injuries can develop into a complex regional pain syndrome. Continuous indwelling sciatic, femoral, and epidural catheters are the mainstays of initial pain management. The pain service may need to combine narcotics, neuroleptic agents, and anti-inflammatory medications during the reconstruction to achieve pain relief, particularly if nerve injury has occurred.

As in prior conflicts, casualties experience a great deal of psychologic trauma. Psychiatric service involvement is essential. During the initial hospitalizations, flashbacks and "animated" wakings from anesthesia may occur. The symptoms of post-traumatic stress syndrome often develop following discharge from the hospital. A large percentage of service members experience sleepless nights, emotional volatility, anger, and flashbacks. Surveying their psychologic status is a routine part of an orthopedic surgery follow-up visit. The war on terrorism is the first major modern American conflict in which large numbers of female service members have been injured in combat, and the nature of their post-traumatic stress may be different when compared with that of male service members.

Summary

Extremity trauma secondary to explosive devices is the most common injury incurred on the contemporary battlefield. Limb salvage is a viable alternative for the treatment of severe open fractures of the lower extremity created by blast injuries. For unilateral injuries, amputation may create a more functional outcome than limb salvage, especially when the open fractures are accompanied by significant soft tissue defects. Limb salvage requires a multidisciplinary effort to reduce complications and maximize success. New fixation devices and bone stimulating factors improve the ability to achieve bone union. The eradication of infection and reconstruction of compromised soft tissues remain the major obstacles to achieving superior functional outcomes. External ring fixators, such as the TSF, show great promise as the definitive fixation for blast fractures and as a reconstructive tool for dealing with residual soft tissue and bone defects.

References

[1] United States Department of Defense. Press resources. Available at: http://www.defenselink. mil/news/casualty.pdf. Accessed September 6, 2005.
[2] Covey DC. Blast and fragment injuries of the musculoskeletal system. J Bone Joint Surg 2002;84-A(7):1221–34.
[3] Patel TH, Wenner KA, Price SA, et al. A US Army Forward Surgical Team's experience in Operation Iraqi Freedom. J Trauma 2004;57(2):201–7.
[4] Lin DL, Kirk KL, Murphy KP, et al. Evaluation of orthopaedic injuries in Operation Enduring Freedom. J Orthop Trauma 2004;18(5):300–5.

[5] London PS. Medical lessons from the Falkland Islands' campaign. Report of a meeting of the United Services Section of the Royal Society of Medicine held at the Royal College of Surgeons on February 17 and 18, 1983. J Bone Joint Surg Br 1983;65:507–10.

[6] Batinica J, Batinica S. War wounds in the Sibenik area during the 1991–1992 war against Croatia. Mil Med 1995;160:124–8.

[7] Mabry RL, Holcomb JB, Baker AM, et al. United States Army Rangers in Somalia: an analysis of combat casualties on an urban battlefield. J Trauma 2000;49(3):515–28.

[8] Gofrit ON, Leibovici D, Shapira SC, et al. The trimodal death distribution of trauma victims: military experience from the Lebanon war. Mil Med 1997;162(1):24–6.

[9] Islinger RB, Kuklo TR, McHale KA. A review of orthopedic injuries in three recent US military conflicts. Mil Med 2000;165(6):463–5.

[10] Elton RC. Orthopaedic war surgery, 85th evacuation hospital, Viet Nam 1968. J Bone Joint Surg Am 1971;53:1231.

[11] Langworthy MJ, Smith JM, Gould M. Treatment of the mangled lower extremity after a terrorist blast injury. Clin Orthop 2004;422:88–96.

[12] Peleg K, Aharonson-Daniel L, Stein M, et al. Gunshot and explosion injuries, characteristics, outcomes, and implications for care of terror-related injuries in Israel. Ann Surg 2004;239(3): 311–8.

[13] Scope A, Farkash U, Lynn M, et al. Mortality epidemiology in low-intensity warfare: Israel Defense Forces' experience. Injury 2001;32(1):1–3.

[14] Hamilton FH. A practical treatise on military surgery and hygiene. New York: Balleire Brothers; 1861. p. 165–83.

[15] Van der Meij WKN. No leg to stand on: historical relation between amputation surgery and prostheseology. Turnhout (Belgium): Proost International Book Production; 1995.

[16] Bohne WHO. Atlas of amputation surgery. Stuttgart (Germany): Georg Thieme Verlag; 1987.

[17] Kay HW, Newman JD. Relative incidences of new amputations. Orthotics Prosthetics 1975; 29:3–16.

[18] Anderson R. Automatic method for the treatment of fractures of the tibia and fibula. SGO 1934;58:639–46.

[19] Hoffman R. 'Rotules a os' pour la 'reduction dirigee, non sanglante des fractures' ('Osteotaxis'). Helvetic Medica Acta 1938;5:844–50.

[20] Board for the Study of the Severely Wounded. The physiologic effects of wounds. Washington (DC): The Office of the Surgeon General, Department of the Army; 1952.

[21] Hughes WC. Arterial repair during the Korean War. Ann Surg 1958;147:555–61.

[22] Artz CP, Howard JM, Sako Y, et al. Clinical experiences in the early management of the most severely injured battle casualties. Ann Surg 1955;141(3):285–96.

[23] Brisbin RL, Geib PO, Eiseman B. Secondary disruption of vascular repair following war wounds. Arch Surg 1969;99(6):787–91.

[24] Rich NM, Baugh JH, Hughes CW. Popliteal artery injuries in Vietnam. Am J Surg 1969;118: 531–4.

[25] DeBakey ME, Simeone FA. Battle injuries of the arteries in World War II, an analysis of 2471 cases. Ann Surg 1946;123:534–79.

[26] Zipperman HH. The management of soft tissue missile wounds in war and peace. J Trauma 1961;1:361–7.

[27] Ziv I, Mosheiff R, Zeligowski A, et al. Crush injuries of the foot with compartment syndrome: immediate one-stage management. Foot Ankle 1989;9(4):185–9.

[28] Lange RH, Bach AW, Hansen ST. Open tibia fractures with associated vascular injuries: prognosis for limb salvage. J Trauma 1985;25:203–8.

[29] Hansen ST. The type IIIC tibial fracture: salvage or amputation? J Bone Joint Surg Am 1987; 69:799–800.

[30] Drost TF, Rosemurgy AS, Proctor D. Outcome of treatment of combined orthopedic and arterial trauma to the lower extremity. J Trauma 1989;29:1331–4.

[31] Caudle RJ, Stern PJ. Severe open fractures of the tibia. J Bone Joint Surg Am 1987;69:801–7.

[32] Swiontkowski MF, MacKenzie EJ, Bosse MJ, et al. Factors influencing the decision to amputate or reconstruct after high-energy lower-extremity trauma. J Trauma 2002;52(4):641–9.

[33] Deffer PA, Moll JH, LaNoue AM. The Ertl osteoplastic below-knee amputation: Proceedings of the American Academy of Orthopaedic Surgeons. J Bone Joint Surg Am 1971;53:1028.

[34] Pinto MA, Harris WW. Fibular segment bone bridging in trans-tibial amputation. Prosthet Orthot Int 2004;28(3):220–4.

[35] Dougherty PJ. Transtibial amputees from the Vietnam War: twenty-eight-year follow-up. J Bone Joint Surg Am 2001;83-A(3):383–9.

[36] Anglen JO. Comparison of soap and antibiotic solutions for irrigation of lower-limb open fracture wounds. J Bone Joint Surg Am 2005;87:1415–22.

[37] Kingsley A. The wound infection continuum and its application to clinical practice. Ostomy Wound Manage 2003;49(7A suppl):1–7.

[38] Robson MC. Wound infection: a failure of wound healing caused by an imbalance of bacteria. Surg Clin North Am 1997;77:637–50.

[39] Valenziano CP, Chattar-Cora D, O'Neill A, et al. Efficacy of primary wound cultures in long bone open extremity fractures: are they of any value? Arch Orthop Trauma Surg 2002;122(5):259–61.

[40] Kreder HJ, Armstrong P. The significance of perioperative cultures in open pediatric lower extremity fractures. Clin Orthop 1994;302:206–12.

[41] Pruitt Jr BA, McManus AT, Kim SH, et al. Burn wound infections: current status. World J Surg 1998;22:135–45.

[42] Lawrence JC. The bacteriology of burns. J Hosp Infect 1985;6:3–17.

[43] Centers for Disease Control and Prevention (CDC). Acinetobacter baumannii infections among patients at military medical facilities treating injured US service members, 2002–2004. MMWR Morb Mortal Wkly Rep 2004;53(45):1063–6.

[44] Davis KA, Moran KA, McAllister CK, et al. Multidrug-resistant Acinetobacter extremity infections in soldiers. Emerg Infect Dis 2005;11(8):1218–24.

[45] Wahlig H, Dingeldein E, Bergmann R, et al. The release of gentamycin from polymethylmethacrylate beads: an experimental and pharmacokinetic study. J Bone Joint Surg Br 1978;60:270–5.

[46] Evans RP, Nelson CL. Gentamicin-impregnated polymethylmethacrylate beads compared with systemic antibiotic therapy in the treatment of chronic osteomyelitis. Clin Orthop 1993;295:37–42.

[47] Salvati EA, Callahan JJ. Reimplantation in infection: elution of gentamycin from cement and beads. Clin Orthop 1986;207:89–93.

[48] Walenkamp GH, Kleijn LL, de Leeuw M. Osteomyelitis treated with gentamycin-PMMA beads: 100 patients followed for 1–12 years. Acta Orthop Scand 1998;69(5):518–22.

[49] Mader JT, Calhoun J, Cobos J. In vitro evaluation of antibiotic diffusion from antibiotic-impregnated biodegradable beads and polymethylmethacrylate beads. Antimicrob Agents Chemother 1997;41(2):415–8.

[50] Haydon MD, Blaha DJ, Mancinelli C, et al. Audiometric thresholds in osteomyelitis patients treated with gentamycin-impregnated methylmethacrylate beads (Septopal). Clin Orthop 1993;295:43–6.

[51] Roeder B, Van Gils CC, Maling S. Antibiotic beads in the treatment of diabetic pedal osteomyelitis. J Foot Ankle Surg 2000;39(2):124–30.

[52] Calhoun JH, Klemm K, Anger DM, et al. Use of antibiotic-PMMA beads in the ischemic foot. Orthopedics 1994;17(5):453–8.

[53] Myerson MS, Miller SD, Henderson M, et al. Staged arthrodesis for salvage of the septic hallux metatarsophalangeal joint. Clin Orthop 1994;307:174–81.

[54] Penner MJ, Duncan CP, Masri BA. The in vitro elution characteristics of antibiotic-loaded CMW and Palacos-R bone cements. J Arthroplasty 1999;14(2):209–14.

[55] Stevens CM, Tetsworth KD, Calhoun JH, et al. An articulated antibiotic spacer used for infected total knee arthroplasty: a comparative in vitro elution study of Simplex and Palacos bone cements. J Orthop Res 2005;23(1):27–33.

[56] Merkhan IK, Hasenwinkel JM, Gilbert JL. Gentamicin release from two-solution and powder-liquid poly(methyl methacrylate)-based bone cements by using novel pH method. J Biomed Mater Res 2004;69(3):577–83.

[57] Greene N, Holtom PD, Warren CA, et al. In vitro elution of tobramycin and vancomycin poly-methylmethacrylate beads and spacers from Simplex and Palacos. Am J Orthop 1998;27(3): 201–5.

[58] Ragel CV, Vallet-Regi M. In vitro bioactivity and gentamycin release from glass-polymer-antibiotic composites. J Biomed Mater Res 2000;51(3):424–9.

[59] Becker PL, Smith RA, Dutkowsky JP, et al. Comparison of antibiotic release from poly-methymethacrylate beads and sponge collagen. J Orthop Res 1994;12(5):737–41.

[60] Calhoun JH, Mader JT. Treatment of osteomyelitis with a biodegradable antibiotic implant. Clin Orthop 1997;341:206–14.

[61] Del Real RP, Padilla S, Vallet-Regi M. Gentamicin release from hydroxyapatite/poly(ethyl methacrylate)/poly(methylmethacrylate) composites. J Biomed Mater Res 2000;52:1–7.

[62] Breidenbach WC, Trager S. Quantitative culture technique and infection in complex wounds of the extremities closed with free flaps. Plast Reconstr Surg 1995;95:860–5.

[63] Godina M. Early microsurgical reconstruction of complex trauma of the extremities. Plast Reconstr Surg 1986;78:285–92.

[64] Byrd HS, Spicer TE, Cierny G, Tebbets JB. Management of open tibial fractures. Plast Reconstr Surg 1985;76:719–30.

[65] Lebeeu F, Pasuch M, Toussain P, et al. External fixation in war traumatology: report from the Rwandese War (October 1, 1990 to August 1, 1993). J Trauma Injury Infection Critical Care 1996;40(3):S223–8.

[66] Nemec B, Santic V, Matovinovic D, et al. War wounds to the foot. Mil Med 1999;165(1):18–9.

[67] Chambers LW, Rhee P, Baker BC, et al. Initial experience of US Marine Corps forward resuscitative surgical system during Operation Iraqi Freedom. Arch Surg 2005;140:26–32.

[68] Carey ME. Analysis of wounds incurred by US Army Seventh Corps of Personnel treated in Corps hospitals during Operation Desert Storm, February 20 to March 10, 1991. J Trauma Injury Infection Critical Care 1996;40(3):S165–9.

[69] Hammer RR, Rooser B, Lidman D, et al. Simplified external fixation for primary management of severe musculoskeletal injuries under war and peace time conditions. J Orthop Trauma 1996; 8:545–54.

[70] Davila S, Mikulic D. War injuries to the talus. Mil Med 2000;166(8):705–70.

[71] Ilizarov GA. The principles of the Ilizarov method. Bull Hosp Jt Dis 1988;48:1–11.

[72] Pommer A, Muhr G, David A. Hydroxyapatite-coated Schanz pins in external fixators used for distraction osteogenesis: a randomized, controlled trial. J Bone Joint Surg Am 2002;84(7): 1162–6.

[73] Piza G, Caja VL, Gonzalez-Viejo MA, et al. Hydroxyapatite-coated external-fixation pins: the effect on pin loosening and pin-track infection in leg lengthening for short stature. J Bone Joint Surg Br 2004;86(6):892–7.

[74] BESST Study Group. Recombinant human bone morphogenetic protein-2 for treatment of open tibial fractures. J Bone Joint Surg Am 2002;84:2123–34.

ELSEVIER
SAUNDERS

Foot Ankle Clin N Am
11 (2006) 183–190

FOOT AND
ANKLE CLINICS

Treatment of Posttraumatic Injuries to the Nerves in the Foot and Ankle

Mark A. Glazebrook, MD, MSc, PhD[a],*, Justin L. Paletz, MD[b]

[a]Division of Orthopedic Surgery, Queen Elizabeth II Health Sciences Center, Halifax Infirmary,
(Suite 4867), Dalhousie University, 1796 Summer Street, Halifax, Nova Scotia B3H 3A7, Canada
[b]Division of Plastic Surgery, Queen Elizabeth II Health Sciences Center, Halifax Infirmary,
(Suite 4445), Dalhousie University, 1796 Summer Street, Halifax, Nova Scotia B3H 3A7, Canada

Injuries to the nerves of the foot and ankle may present with a varying degree of clinical consequences, depending on the type, location, and extent of injuries. Clinical consequences may range from minor pain and numbness, such as experienced with small distal nerves (eg, Morton's neuroma), or more significant clinical consequences, such as neurogenic pain and loss of motor function that are experienced with injuries to large nerves more proximal in the leg.

The type of injury to a nerve may be classified as primary or secondary (Box 1). Primary nerve injuries are diagnosed easily and result from direct trauma, such as lacerations or a crush injury. Secondary nerve injuries result from pathologic processes that cause subsequent injury to a nerve. Secondary injuries include systemic disease or local tumor, which causes a compression nerve injury.

Primary injuries are diagnosed easily but the extent of injury must be understood to predict prognosis and guide treatment. Primary injuries that cause conduction block, but leave the nerve intact, are called neurapraxias and have the best prognosis for recovery. A primary nerve injury that results in a divided nerve (neurotemesis) has less potential for recovery. The nerve injuries that cause division with extensive crush and widespread damage leave surgery as the only

* Corresponding author.
E-mail address: markglazebr@ns.sympatico.ca (M.A. Glazebrook).

Box 1. Etiologic classification of different types of injuries to the nerves in the foot and ankle

Primary

    Laceration
    Crush
    Traction

Secondary

    Tumor
    Compartment syndrome
    Deformity
    Constriction
    Systemic disease
    Fracture

---

option for recovery. It is important to understand the mechanism and extent of injury to appreciate the treatment options and prognosis.

Lastly, location of the nerve injury is important because an understanding of the anatomy of the injured nerve dictates the resultant clinical consequences. Thus, a detailed description of the anatomy and a description of motor and sensory function deserve review (Table 1).

Table 1
Anatomy of the nerves in the foot and ankle

Nerve	Sensory innervation	Motor innervation
Tibial nerve		
Medial plantar nerve	Medial plantar arch 3½ digits	AbH., FHB, FDB, first lumbrical
Lateral plantar nerve	Lateral plantar midfoot 1½ digits	QP, interossi, AddH, ADM, second through fourth lumbricals
Superficial peroneal nerve		
Dorsal intermed. branch	Dorsolateral foot	None
Dorsal medial branch	Dorsomedial foot	None
Deep peroneal nerve	First dorsal webspace	EDB & EHB
Saphenous nerve	Medial hind & midfoot	None
Sural nerve	Lateral border	None

Abbreviations: Abh, abductor hallucis; AddH, adductor hallucis; ADM, adductor digiti minimi; EDB, extensor digitorum brevis; EHB, extensor hallucis brevis; FDB, flexor digitorum brevis; FHB, flexor hallucis brevis; QP, quadratus plantii.

Anatomy

The tibial nerve provides motor and sensory innervation to the foot. It begins in the popliteal fossa and courses through the posterior compartment of the lower leg, posterior to the tibialis posterior muscle. It passes behind the medial malleolus and divides into smaller branches. These branches are the medial plantar nerve, which provides sensation to the medial plantar arch and the medial three and one half digits. The lateral plantar nerve provides sensation to the lateral plantar midfoot and the remaining lateral one and one half digits. The motor component of the medial plantar nerve includes the abductor hallucis, the flexor hallucis brevis, the flexor digitorum brevis, and the first lumbrical. The lateral plantar nerve innervates the quadratus plantae, interossei, abductor hallucis, abductor digiti minimi, and the second to fourth lumbricals.

The medial calcaneal branch of the tibial nerve provides sensation to the plantar aspect of the foot at the heel.

The deep peroneal nerve also provides sensory and motor innervation. The sensory innervation includes the first dorsal web space, whereas the motor innervation includes the extensor digitorum brevis and the extensor hallucis brevis.

The superficial peroneal nerve is a sensory nerve to the foot. It has a dorsal intermediate branch, which provides sensation to the dorsal lateral portion of the foot, and the dorsal medial branch, which supplies sensation to the dorsal medial portion of the foot.

The saphenous nerve is a sensory nerve and it provides sensation to the medial hind and midfoot.

The sural nerve provides sensation to the lateral border of the foot, including its lateral calcaneal branch, which provides sensation to the lateral plantar hindfoot.

History and physical examination

A detailed discussion of the method of injury should take place. This allows assessment of the type, location, and extent of injury. For example, the nerve may have been injured by a sharp, clean laceration or a crush injury from blunt trauma. This dictates the potential for recovery and assists in determining the type of surgical repair that is necessary. A detailed history regarding the nature of the pain experienced is important. If pain is experienced in a particular nerve distribution and is described as sharp, burning, or radiating, then a nerve injury is part of the principal diagnosis. Reports of numbness and lack of sensation or motor function lead the clinician to the appropriate diagnosis.

It also is important to gather a history for the timing of the pain. If there was no obvious injury identified, then the nerve injury could result from a chronic compartment syndrome or an underlying tumor. Nerve injuries from a chronic compartment syndrome characteristically are symptomatic with increased repetitive exercise, whereas a secondary nerve injury from a tumor may cause pain at rest because of the external compression. In a similar way, a Morton's neuroma causes pain secondary to the trauma of compression of a shoe with a tight toe box.

Inquiries about proximal nerve pathology, such as those arising from the central nervous system or systemic illness that may cause nerve injuries (eg, diabetes mellitus), should be made.

When performing a physical examination, the examiner should define the location and extent of injury. While assessing the clinical manifestations of a suspected nerve injury, one must do a detailed sensory and motor examination. If there is a questionable sensory nerve injury, one should perform a detailed sensory testing, including monofilament examination, two-point discrimination in the zone of injury, sharp and dull sensation, and vibration sense. Two-point discrimination in the foot is different from the upper extremity with less precision in discriminating smaller distances. If there is no sensory change and there are nerve symptoms, a Tinel's sign may assist in determining the area of injury.

Changes of skin color, temperature, and swelling also may assist in a diagnosis of chronic regional pain syndrome (reflex sympathetic dystrophy), which is a more ominous diagnosis. Local masses near nerves deserve a work-up to distinguish common benign tumors from less common malignant tumors.

In summary, a sound knowledge of the anatomy of the nerves, together with a detailed history and physical examination, provides an accurate diagnosis of nerve injuries and provides further options for nonoperative and operative treatment.

Investigations

For primary injuries to the nerves of the foot and ankle, a careful clinical history and physical examination usually provide an accurate diagnosis. Secondary injuries to the nerves of a more chronic nature may require electrical nerve conduction studies (ENCSs) to assist with detailing the extent, type, and location of the nerve injury. ENCSs also are useful to follow the recovery of an injured nerve.

If a tumor is included in the differential diagnosis, MRI studies are useful to assist with tumor diagnosis and the anatomic relationship of the tumor to the injured nerve.

Treatment

The ideal treatment for a lacerated nerve is primary repair using epineurial sutures under appropriate magnification. With late presentation, and in secondary nerve injury of the foot and ankle, this often is not possible. Treatment in these situations is determined by the patient's pathology. Symptoms could include pain, sensory loss, or loss of intrinsic muscle function. Sensory loss on the dorsum of the foot and the plantar aspect of the forefoot and toes usually does not result in a significant functional deficit. Loss of sensation on the entire sole of the foot frequently leads to chronic ulceration that is extremely difficult to cure if the sensory deficit cannot be improved. In cases where pain is the dominant presenting symptom, initial treatment often is conservative. Modalities include desensitization of painful scars and neuromata, transcutaneous electrical nerve stimulation, and custom footwear or orthoses to offload the painful area of the foot or ankle. If this approach is unsuccessful, surgery should be considered for the painful neuroma.

Tibial nerve

The tibial nerve provides sensation to most of the sole of the foot, and innervation to most of the intrinsic muscles of the foot, with the exception of the extensor digitorum brevis and the extensor hallucis brevis (see Table 1). An insensate sole, along with loss of the plantar arch secondary to intrinsic muscle paralysis, is tolerated poorly and frequently results in skin breakdown and ulceration. Therefore, continuity of the tibial nerve should be restored whenever possible, even if nerve grafting is required. If a nerve graft is required, the contralateral sural nerve is recommended. The intact ipsilateral sural nerve may provide some neurotization to the insensate area, and further desensitization of an already injured limb should be avoided.

In an acute situation, the lacerated tibial nerve typically can be approximated primarily. Use of an operating microscope may facilitate this. Because this is a mixed motor and sensory nerve, an attempt to align the nerve ends correctly should be attempted. Small vessels on the surface of the proximal and distal nerve can be lined up. In addition, groups of fascicules that match in the transected nerve ends can be used as a guide for proper nerve alignment. Again, however, only epineurial sutures are used.

In chronic injuries, the divided nerve ends frequently cannot be approximated; even with adequate mobilization of the nerve, a reversed sural nerve graft is used. More than one segment of sural nerve may be required to cover the cross-sectional area of exposed tibial nerve ends adequately. The proximal and distal neuromata must be resected. This is continued with the proximal nerve end in a sequential fashion until healthy appearing, unscarred nerve fascicles are apparent. Hattrup and Wood [1] reported that better results were obtained with shorter nerve grafts in comparison with long grafts.

Tibial nerve branches

Division of the medial calcaneal branch of the tibial nerve results in loss of sensation on the heel pad. If sensation remains intact in the remainder of the foot, this usually is not a functional problem. If the transected calcaneal nerve results in a painful neuroma, the neuroma can be resected more proximally, which removes the neuroma from repetitive contact from weight bearing [2].

Laceration of a nerve on the sole of the foot can result in sensory loss, or a painful neuroma. The more distal the injury, the smaller and less functionally significant is the area of sensory loss. If the medial or lateral plantar nerves are divided, they should be repaired primarily, if possible. Positioning an operating microscope to repair nerve injuries that involve the sole of the foot can be difficult, and the patient needs to be in the prone position. If loupe magnification is used, the prone position usually is not necessary. Isolated injury to a common or proper digital nerve usually is tolerated well without repair. Injury to multiple adjacent digital nerves obviously increases the area of sensory loss, and may merit repair. Even if there is little sensory recovery, direct or nerve graft reapproximation of the nerve ends should decrease painful neuroma formation. If repair is not practical, a painful neuroma on the sole of the foot can be re-excised more proximally, or the nerve end can be moved to a more protected position in the foot (eg, intermetatarsal space).

Sural nerve

Frequently, the sural nerve is harvested as a graft for nerve reconstruction procedures. Typically, the resulting sensory loss along the lateral border of the foot is of little functional consequence. Sural nerve injuries may occur secondary to lacerations or crush injuries of the heel or ankle, or iatrogenically (eg, during reconstruction of the lateral ligament of the ankle). In an acute situation, epineurial repair of the nerve is recommended if possible. In cases of a chronic, painful neuroma, the nerve can be transected proximal to the ankle to relocate the neuroma away from repetitive pressure [2,3].

Superficial peroneal nerve

The superficial peroneal nerve exits the deep fascia at about the junction of the middle and distal thirds of the leg. It divides into two branches: the dorsal medial cutaneous nerve and the dorsal intermediate cutaneous nerve. These branches supply sensation to most of the dorsum of the foot and toes. The superficial peroneal nerve can be injured during surgery on the lateral aspect of the ankle and during fasciotomy of the lateral compartment. If recognized acutely, the divided nerve should be repaired.

In chronic situations where a painful neuroma of this nerve exists, nerve repair typically is not possible, and nerve grafting usually is not warranted because the sensory deficit is well tolerated. The neuroma can be transected proximally in the leg to relieve it from contact with footwear and constant movement. If this simple procedure fails, the nerve can be transected more proximally and allowed to retract under the deep fascia [3].

Deep peroneal nerve

This nerve supplies sensation to the first web space dorsally, and motor innervation to the extensor digitorum brevis and the extensor hallucis brevis muscles. Loss of function of this nerve can result in mild weakness of toe extension. Recommendations for treating painful neuromata of this nerve on the dorsum of the foot include dividing the nerve proximally and burying the nerve end in the anterior compartment [2] of the leg, or excising the nerve under the cover of the extensor hallucis brevis muscle [3].

Saphenous nerve

This nerve travels adjacent to the greater saphenous vein, which makes it susceptible to injury during vein harvest for coronary artery bypass grafting or stripping of varicose veins. The small area of sensory loss on the medial aspect of the hind and midfoot is not functionally significant; the typical recommended treatment is resection of the neuroma proximal to the ankle joint.

Complications

Nerve injuries in the ankle and foot can result in painful neuromata. Even with appropriate conservative and surgical intervention, chronic pain syndromes can arise. These may take the form of complex regional pain syndrome type I (reflex sympathetic dystrophy) or type II (pain of neurogenic origin or causalgia). These can be extremely debilitating, and there are patients whose lives are dominated by pain. Optimal management of such problems typically requires surgeon, therapist, and a physician who specializes in chronic pain management to work together to facilitate the patient's recovery. Regional sympathetic blocks may be of benefit in patients who have complex regional pain syndrome type I. In patients who have neuropathic pain, tricyclic antidepressants and some of the anticonvulsant drugs can be of benefit.

Summary

Recognition of acute nerve injury in the foot and ankle requires a careful history and physical examination. Lacerations of the tibial nerve or medial plantar or lateral plantar nerve should be repaired primarily, if possible. In chronic cases, repair or reconstruction of the tibial nerve with nerve grafting should be considered. Other types of chronic nerve injury in the foot and ankle should be managed based on clinical assessment. Initial attempts at pain management frequently involve conservative measures. If required, surgery can involve redirection or placement of painful neuromata in areas that are less exposed to repetitive movement and pressure.

References

[1] Hattrup SJ, Wood MB. Delayed neural reconstruction in the lower extremity: results of interfascicular nerve grafting. Foot Ankle 1986;7:105–9.
[2] Thordarson DB, Shean CJ. Nerve and tendon lacerations about the foot and ankle. J Am Acad Orthop Surg 2005;13:186–96.
[3] Gould JS. Complex nerve problems of the foot and ankle. In: Nunley JA, Pfeffer GB, Sanders RW, et al, editors. Advanced reconstruction of the foot and ankle. Rosemont, Illinois: American Academy of Orthopedic Surgeons; 2003. p. 473–9.

ELSEVIER
SAUNDERS

Foot Ankle Clin N Am
11 (2006) 191–201

FOOT AND
ANKLE CLINICS

Reconstruction of the Foot After Leg or Foot Compartment Syndrome

Mark D. Perry, MD[a],*, Arthur Manoli II, MD[b]

[a]Department of Orthopaedic Surgery, University of Texas Southwestern Medical Center,
5323 Harry Hines Boulevard, Dallas, TX 75390-8883, USA
[b]Michigan International Foot and Ankle Center, 44555 Woodward Avenue, Suite 105,
Pontiac, MI 48341, USA

Compartment syndrome has been well recognized as a complication of lower extremity injury. Nevertheless, literature discussing specific reconstructions for compartment syndrome sequelae is scarce [1,2]. Seddon [3] in 1966 described the pathophysiology of lower limb contractures secondary to compartment syndrome, and Manoli and coworkers in 1991 presented their work on the treatment of established ischemic contractures [2].

The pathophysiology of compartment syndrome is well understood. Interestingly, upper limb ischemic contracture occurs owing to a different mechanism than lower limb injury. Compartment syndrome in the upper limb tends to develop from a vascular insult of the brachial artery, which results in predictable ischemia distally [3]. Lower limb compartment syndrome is often associated with a fracture or a crush type injury. These tissues experience not only ischemia from increased compartment pressures but also a direct crush injury resulting in cellular damage [4]. Elevation ischemia intraoperatively or from high postoperative leg elevation is an increasing cause of compartment syndrome.

The authors do not have any commercial or proprietary interest in any equipment mentioned in this article.

* Corresponding author.
E-mail address: Mark.Perry@UTSouthwestern.edu (M.D. Perry).

Prevention

Despite the increasing vigilance in the orthopedic community to diagnosis compartment syndrome, it is still an often preventable but dreaded complication [5]. Compartment syndrome must be recognized and "fixed" by treating it acutely. Avoidance of the problem leads to catastrophic late complications. The physician must perform an honest assessment evaluating the empirical and clinical evidence [6]. Denial of compartment syndrome is never appropriate treatment.

Polytrauma patients see multiple physicians [7] who subsequently run many tests [8] and perform multiple evaluations [9], increasing the chance of failed communication resulting in a critical delay in diagnosis. Failing to make a diagnosis of compartment syndrome is the most common treatment error [10,11]. Clinical judgment unfortunately is inaccurate, and only dramatic compartment syndromes are easily evident. The "subtle" compartment syndromes are the most difficult to define, resulting in significant deformities and late complications.

The diagnosis of compartment syndrome should be suspected in many clinical settings [12–18]. Orthopedic surgeons should have a high degree of suspicion when treating fractures of the tibial shaft and tibial plateau, high-energy ankle injuries, and pilon fractures. Fractures of the femur and the foot can also result in compartment syndrome. Knee dislocations and vascular bypass surgery can result in compartment syndrome from prolonged vascular compromise and reperfusion. Transplant surgery and cardiac bypass surgery can cause compartment syndrome from prolonged hypotension. Infections and circumferential burns are also known to provide increased compartment pressures. Drug overdose and prolonged pressure can cause compartment syndromes in unusual locations. Prolonged limb elevation during urologic, general, transplant, and orthopedic surgery can result in muscle damage and compartment syndrome during reperfusion. Unusual conditions causing compartment syndrome include hemophilia and snake bites.

Leg compartment syndrome late sequelae occur secondary to a delay in diagnosis or to inadequate decompression. Orthopedic surgeons and general surgeons can treat acute compartment syndrome of the leg. Depending on the training of the surgeon, the release may be inadequate. Fig. 1 shows the leg of a patient whose fasciotomy performed by a nonorthopedic service for compartment syndrome was done too high, missing the posterior compartment. The deep posterior compartment was never released, resulting in a severe deformity; however, the patient achieved a plantigrade foot with relatively good function following scarred muscle excision and a midfoot osteotomy.

Fig. 2 illustrates another error during fasciotomies. Although the compartments were released, the skin bridge anteriorly was too small and necrosed. Subsequently, the patient's large anterior wound prevented internal fixation of his bimalleolar ankle fracture.

Orthopedic surgeons focus on long skin incisions with direct visualization of the fascia releasing between the intermuscular septae. In addition, four compartment fasciotomies should be performed if lower limb compartment syndrome is

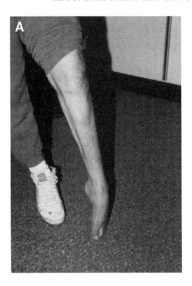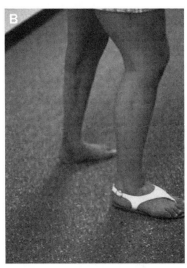

Fig. 1. (*A*) Preoperative and (*B*) postoperative clinical photographs of an untreated deep posterior compartment syndrome. A plantigrade foot was attainable following scarred muscle excision and a midfoot osteotomy.

suspected in a trauma situation. A two-compartment release is appropriate only for nontraumatic, chronic exertional compartment syndrome situations.

Isolated foot compartment syndromes have been described. Late complications include contracture of the quadratus plantae [19,20]. Approximately 10% of intra-articular calcaneal fractures develop foot compartment syndrome [21]. Foot compartment syndrome can also occur after Lisfranc fracture-dislocations, crush injuries, elevation ischemia, and multiple metatarsal fractures. Any time there is a combination of forefoot, midfoot, and hindfoot injury, foot compartment syndrome must be suspected [22–24].

The late foot deficit after foot compartment syndrome includes stiffness and decreased sensation. The lesser toes develop clawing owing to intrinsic muscle

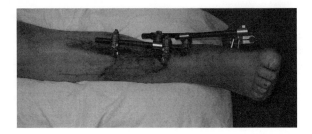

Fig. 2. Photograph demonstrates skin necrosis treated with a split-thickness skin graft after fasciotomy wounds were placed incorrectly.

weakness or contracture, which can be significantly painful. Foot compartments connect between the calcaneal compartment and the deep posterior compartment of the leg [25,26]. Foot compartments should be released to prevent the development of leg compartment syndrome [26]. Some physicians argue that isolated acute foot compartment syndrome should be observed and a late reconstruction performed if necessary.

Delay in diagnosis in the acute phase of care

Patients may present late in the acute phase after the pain has become reduced, indicating the muscle is no longer viable. This "gray area" exists for patients outside of 6 hours of symptoms. If there is an opportunity to prevent compartment syndrome from developing in other compartments, a fasciotomy must be performed. Exposed dead muscle may become infected, potentially leading to below knee amputation despite multiple débridements (Fig. 3).

In patients for whom there is no expectation of salvaging viable muscle after a compartment syndrome, fasciotomy should not be performed. The muscle necrosis will not progress to infection [27] if the skin is intact. If necessary, the patient can be placed temporarily on dialysis during the rhabdomyolysis and the resulting deformity addressed later.

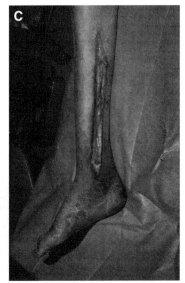
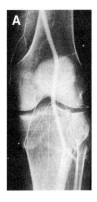
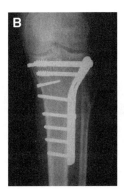

Fig. 3. (*A*) Angiogram showing lateral tibial plateau fracture. (*B*) Internal fixation. (*C*) After multiple débridements, the wound became infected and eventually required a below knee amputation.

Late techniques

Clinically, the diagnosis of deep posterior compartment fibrosis is established by the presence of equinus and cavus with a resulting heel varus and claw toes [25,28]. The goal of reconstruction of the foot is to restore a functional and minimally painful plantigrade foot. The contracture is treated once the deforming forces and scarred muscles have been studied. All fibrotic muscle must be released and excised, because incomplete excision will cause recurrence.

Although rare, an amputation may be indicated because of pain, ulceration, and rigid deformity. Fig. 4 shows the dorsum of the foot of a patient with a closed head injury, a spinal cord injury, and leg compartment syndrome. At the time of presentation, wounds had developed after the patient was pushed in a wheel chair with the ankle in a rigid plantar flexed position. This case illustrates the importance of a neutral ankle position, even in nonambulatory patients. In these patients, the limb can be salvaged by appropriate releases or transfers, preserving patient body image, acting as a counterweight for wheelchair sitting, and assisting in transfers.

Although compartment syndrome can affect all compartments, the resulting deformity depends on the degree of involvement and the anatomy of the muscles affected. Although an anterior compartment syndrome may result in loss of active ankle dorsiflexion, this may not cause a functional deformity. Passive stretching during sleep may maintain motion. An isolated posterior compartment syndrome involving the flexor hallucis longus (FHL) or posterior tibial tendon may cause a significant deformity owing to a lack of antagonistic muscle contraction and strength of the anterior compartment.

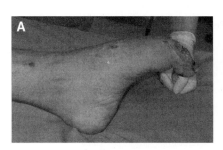
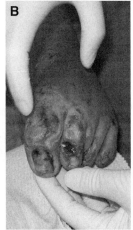

Fig. 4. Toe ulcers. (*A*) Lateral and (*B*) anteroposterior photographs following nontreatment of post compartment syndrome deformity.

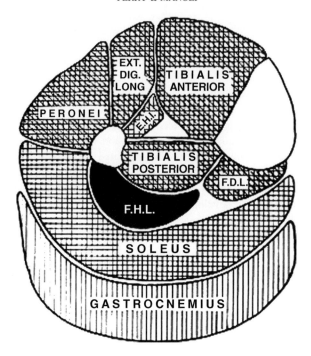

Fig. 5. Diagram showing vulnerability to ischemia of muscles of the leg. The flexor hallucis longus is the most frequently damaged, but the interior muscles, which are superficial, suffer considerably. (*From* Seddon HJ. Volkmann's ischaemia in the lower limb. J Bone Joint Surg Br 1966; 48(4):627–36; with permission.) © British Editorial Society of Bone and Joint Surgery.

The posterior compartment is the most likely to cause late symptoms (Fig. 5). Over 60% of Seddon's subjects had FHL involvement, with the tibialis posterior and the flexor digitorum longus having 40% involvement. In contrast, the gastrocnemius (20%) and the soleus (25%) were less affected [3].

Fig. 6 shows the leg of an intensive care unit patient in whom systemic inflammatory response syndrome (SIRS) and compartment syndrome developed.

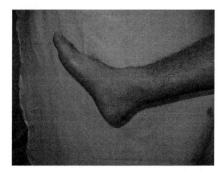

Fig. 6. A deformity of plantar flexion without inversion occurs when the deep compartment is spared.

Releases were performed, and 6 months later, the patient still had residual deformity. The ankle was fixed in 20 degrees of plantar flexion without varus position of the foot. The calf was rigid to palpation. The patient developed fibrosis of the soleus muscle, without involvement of the deep posterior compartment.

Contracture of the deep posterior compartment causes the typical late appearance of leg compartment syndrome. The foot is held internally rotated and in a cavus position with the heel in corresponding varus. Release of the Achilles tendon alone will not correct this deformity; instead, the ischemic muscle should be excised to correct the foot position and prevent recurrence.

Fig. 7 demonstrates the recurrence of deformity after tenotomy treatment. This 47-year-old woman developed compartment syndrome as a complication of a vascular procedure. Despite acute fasciotomies, late deformity developed. In the operating room, it was determined that a posterior release of the Achilles tendon resolved all but 10 degrees of plantar flexion. A tenotomy of the posterior tibial tendon was also performed to place the ankle in a neutral position. Despite postoperative placement in an ankle foot orthosis, after 16 months, a rigid equinus deformity recurred.

Patients with a cavus foot secondary to compartment syndrome also present with a significant internal rotation of the foot and a varus heel. The patient will correct this deformity by externally rotating at the hip. Some of the patients in the study by Manoli and coworkers [2] were previously recommended to undergo rotational osteotomies of this deformity because of the believed internal rotation of the fracture at the deformity site.

Occasionally, an early release of the claw toes via tenotomy may be performed to prevent further development of deformity. A heel cord lengthening or slide may prevent a major equinus component from developing. During late surgical reconstruction, muscle excision, release of contracted joint capsules and tissue, as well as osteotomies and fusions may be required to achieve a plantigrade foot [29].

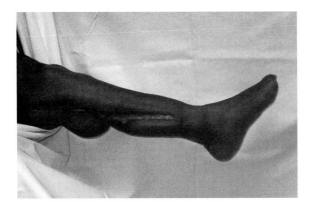

Fig. 7. Photograph shows recurrence following tenotomy without scarred muscle excision.

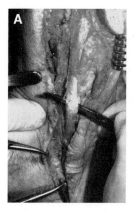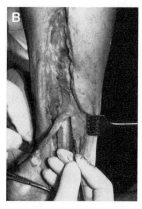

Fig. 8. (*A*) Testing a tendon for excursion and (*B*) excising the fibrotic components.

Exploration of the compartments requires good visualization. Each tendon must be checked for excursion individually (Fig. 8). Any tendon without excursion must have all nonviable muscle removed. A first metatarsal osteotomy and a calcaneal osteotomy can correct heel varus [30].

Claw toes that develop from foot compartment syndrome may require proximal interphalangeal (PIP) joint resections (Fig. 9). The contracted flexor tendon may lack excursion, preventing a functional flexor to extensor tendon transfer [29]. If flexible but tight, the flexor tendon should be taken as far distal to the PIP as possible to have enough length to transfer to the base of the proximal phalanx.

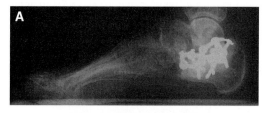

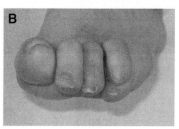

Fig. 9. (*A*) A displaced intra-articular calcaneal fracture that did not undergo fasciotomy for foot compartment syndrome. (*B*) Rigid claw toes that subsequently developed.

Following débridement of ischemic muscle, the surgical wounds are closed over a drain to prevent hematoma [2]. These limbs have undergone significant trauma, and skin problems can occur after late reconstructions. Great care needs to be taken in handling the soft tissue envelope during reconstruction. Patients are kept in a cast and encouraged to weight bear as tolerated. Casting holds the ankle in a neutral position during recovery. If bony work such as subtalar fusion, triple arthrodesis, or osteotomy has been performed, weight bearing should be delayed while the ankle is splinted. Early weight bearing will assist dorsiflexion.

In situations where a tremendous deformity exits, or in a setting of a poor tissue envelope, initial correction may be achieved with an external frame (Fig. 10). A percutaneous tendo-Achilles lengthening and incremental adjustment will allow the foot to be placed under the leg with minimal surgical morbidity. At the authors' center, a multiplanar frame has been used to correct ischemic contractures 1 and 2 years post injury. The frame concurrently corrects the plantar flexion and the varus deformity. Current results for a patient at 1 year and for another at 6 months postoperatively have revealed no deformity or recurrence.

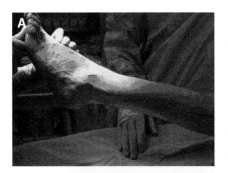
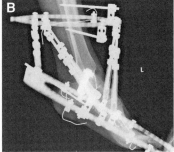
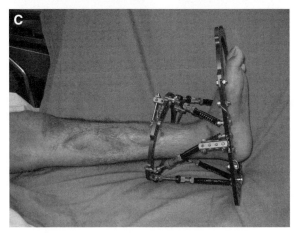

Fig. 10. (*A*) Preoperative maximal passive dorsiflexion. (*B*) Application of frame. (*C*) Correction after incremental changes over 2 months.

External fixation was continued for 3 months following deformity correction. Once the foot was in a position allowing weight bearing (plantar flexion of approximately 20 degrees), a custom footplate was attached to the frame. Lymphedema may occur during the deformity correction secondary to compression of the sinus tarsi. If lymphedema suddenly develops, the frame is adjusted to relax the deformity, and the desired position is achieved at a slower rate. In these cases, once the ankle is in a functional position, the patient may be followed clinically and, if necessary, undergo scarred muscle excision in a standard fashion if the deformity starts to recur.

Recurrence is minimized by excising scarred muscle as well as the tendon components. Hansen's group did not find pes planus after posterior tibial excision [2]. The spring ligament should not be disrupted. All viable muscle is kept and may be used for tendon transfers. Clawson's test of the long flexors may not be possible in patients with leg compartment syndrome because of ankle stiffness [31].

Summary

Compartment syndrome should be treated early and aggressively to prevent late complications. Patients may have late deformity because of a failure of diagnosis, inadequate decompression, or a delay in fasciotomies [32]. Late reconstruction will allow a plantigrade and relatively functional foot. Complete excision of scarred muscle will prevent recurrence in established deformities. Early treatment may prevent significant functional impairment by well-placed tenotomies. In patients with severe long-term deformities with extensive soft tissue contraction, incremental correction may be an appropriate intermediate intervention.

References

[1] Santi MD, Botte MJ. Volkmann's ischemic contracture of the foot and ankle: evaluation and treatment of established deformity. Foot Ankle Int 1995;16(6):368–77.
[2] Manoli 2nd A, Smith DG, Hansen Jr ST. Scarred muscle excision for the treatment of established ischemic contracture of the lower extremity. Clin Orthop 1993;292:309–14.
[3] Seddon HJ. Volkmann's ischaemia in the lower limb. J Bone Joint Surg Br 1966;48(4): 627–36.
[4] Kikuchi S, Hasue M, Watanabe M. Ischemic contracture in the lower limb. Clin Orthop 1978; 134:185–92.
[5] Bhattacharyya T, Vrahas MS. The medical-legal aspects of compartment syndrome. J Bone Joint Surg Am 2004;86(4):864–8.
[6] Holden CE. Compartmental syndromes following trauma. Clin Orthop 1975;113:95–102.
[7] Giannoudis PV, Nicolopoulos C, Dinopoulos H, et al. The impact of lower leg compartment syndrome on health related quality of life. Injury 2002;33(2):117–21.
[8] Farrell CM, Rubin DI, Haidukewych GJ. Acute compartment syndrome of the leg following diagnostic electromyography. Muscle Nerve 2003;27(3):374–7.

[9] Cascio BM, Wilckens JH, Ain MC, et al. Documentation of acute compartment syndrome at an academic health-care center. J Bone Joint Surg Am 2005;87(2):346–50.

[10] Richards H, Langston A, Kulkarni R, et al. Does patient controlled analgesia delay the diagnosis of compartment syndrome following intramedullary nailing of the tibia? Injury 2004;35(3): 296–8.

[11] Hope MJ, McQueen MM. Acute compartment syndrome in the absence of fracture. J Orthop Trauma 2004;18(4):220–4.

[12] Ashworth MJ, Patel N. Compartment syndrome following ankle fracture-dislocation: a case report. J Orthop Trauma 1998;12(1):67–8.

[13] Dhawan A, Doukas WC. Acute compartment syndrome of the foot following an inversion injury of the ankle with disruption of the anterior tibial artery: a case report. J Bone Joint Surg Am 2003;85(3):528–32.

[14] Russell Jr GV, Pearsall AW, Caylor MT, et al. Acute compartment syndrome after rupture of the medial head of the gastrocnemius muscle. South Med J 2000;93(2):247–9.

[15] Reuben A, Clouting E. Compartment syndrome after thrombolysis for acute myocardial infarction. Emerg Med J 2005;22(1):77.

[16] Meldrum R, Lipscomb P. Compartment syndrome of the leg after less than 4 hours of elevation on a fracture table. South Med J 2002;95(2):269–71.

[17] Noorpuri BS, Shahane SA, Getty CJ. Acute compartment syndrome following revisional arthroplasty of the forefoot: the dangers of ankle-block. Foot Ankle Int 2000;21(8):680–2.

[18] Mendelson S, Mendelson A, Holmes J. Compartment syndrome after acute rupture of the peroneus longus in a high school football player: a case report. Am J Orthop 2003;32(10):510–2.

[19] Andermahr J, Helling HJ, Rehm KE, et al. The vascularization of the os calcaneum and the clinical consequences. Clin Orthop 1999;363:212–8.

[20] Manoli 2nd A, Weber TG. Fasciotomy of the foot: an anatomical study with special reference to release of the calcaneal compartment. Foot Ankle 1990;10(5):267–75.

[21] Perry MD, Manoli 2nd A. Foot compartment syndrome. Orthop Clin North Am 2001;32(1): 103–11.

[22] Shereff MJ. Compartment syndromes of the foot. Instr Course Lect 1990;39:127–32.

[23] Manoli 2nd A. Compartment syndromes of the foot: current concepts. Foot Ankle 1990;10(6): 340–4.

[24] Fulkerson E, Razi A, Tejwani N. Review: acute compartment syndrome of the foot. Foot Ankle Int 2003;24(2):180–7.

[25] Karlstrom G, Lonnerholm T, Olerud S. Cavus deformity of the foot after fracture of the tibial shaft. J Bone Joint Surg Am 1975;57(7):893–900.

[26] Manoli 2nd A, Fakhouri AJ, Weber TG. Concurrent compartment syndromes of the foot and leg. Foot Ankle 1993;14(6):339–42.

[27] Viau MR, Pedersen HE, Salcicioli GG, et al. Ectopic calcification as a late sequela of compartment syndrome: report of two cases. Clin Orthop 1983;176:178–80.

[28] Matsen III FA, Clawson DK. The deep posterior compartmental syndrome of the leg. J Bone Joint Surg Am 1975;57(1):34–9.

[29] Manoli A. What happens if you do nothing? Presented at the AOFAS 21st Annual Summer Meeting. Boston, July 15–17, 2005.

[30] Younger AS, Hansen Jr ST. Adult cavovarus foot. J Am Acad Orthop Surg 2005;13(5):302–15.

[31] Clawson DK. Claw toes following tibial fracture. Clin Orthop 1974;103:47–8.

[32] Jose RM, Viswanathan N, Aldlyami E, et al. A spontaneous compartment syndrome in a patient with diabetes. J Bone Joint Surg Br 2004;86(7):1068–70.

ELSEVIER
SAUNDERS

Foot Ankle Clin N Am
11 (2006) 203–215

FOOT AND
ANKLE CLINICS

Reconstruction of the Infected Traumatized Joint

Alastair S.E. Younger, MB, ChB, MSc, ChM, FRCSC[a,b,*],
Mark S. Myerson, MD[c]

[a]Department of Orthopaedics, The University of British Columbia, 401-1160 Burrard Street,
Vancouver, British Columbia V6Z 2E8, Canada
[b]British Columbia's Foot and Ankle Clinic, Providence Health Care
[c]Foot and Ankle Service, Department of Orthopaedic Surgery, The Union Memorial Hospital,
Baltimore, MD, USA

In some cases the injured joint has posttraumatic arthritic change, and the surgeon is challenged with known or potential infection that confounds the treatment plan. Failure to treat the associated deep infection adequately results in failure to achieve the surgical goals. Ongoing infection can compromise the soft tissue envelope significantly by sinus tract formation or inflammation. The local bone may be eroded or softened which compromises the reconstructive alternatives. Attempted fusion in the face of undiagnosed and untreated infection may cause the fusion to fail. All of these issues can result in a below-knee amputation (Fig. 1).

Correct management of the infected traumatized joint can prevent these outcomes if the treating surgeon considers the diagnosis and follows the principles that are involved in treatment. The initial phase is to diagnose and investigate the possibility of infection. Before initiating a course of treatment, it is essential to have an appropriate goal for the patient. This goal must be realistic, and in keeping with the patient's needs. Perhaps the worst thing that we can do as surgeons is to embark on a complex course of reconstruction when the patient would benefit from a more timely below-knee amputation. This issue must be broached with patients who have infection of the foot and ankle, particularly

* Corresponding author. 401-1160 Burrard Street, Vancouver, British Columbia V6Z 2E8, Canada.
E-mail address: asyounger@shaw.ca (A.S.E. Younger).

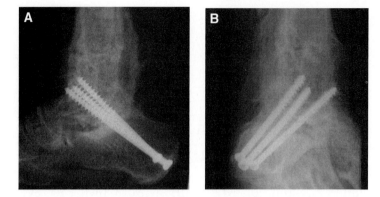

Fig. 1. (*A–B*) A patient with an ankle fusion for work-related posttraumatic arthritis with excision of the fibula. He presented with subtalar arthritis that was treated with a subtalar fusion. He developed a draining nonunion of the subtalar joint. After discussion of the alternatives (free flap and revision subtalar fusion) he elected to undergo a below-knee amputation.

those who have osteomyelitis. This becomes particularly important in the context of the remaining function of the lower extremity, because a patient who has a stiff, functionless foot and ankle with a healed infection may be worse off than a healthy amputee.

History and physical examination

Certain aspects of the history should alert the surgeon to the potential diagnosis of infection. Foot and ankle infections require a portal. Compound injuries are associated with an increased risk for ongoing infection, because a portal for bacterial contamination is created at the time of initial injury [1,2]. Infection risk increases with increased bacterial contamination and is prevented by healthy local tissues. Therefore, infection risk increases with Gustillo grade. Contamination with infected dead material, and a significant delay in debridement affect outcome adversely. Stripping of soft tissues results in loss of local blood supply and deterioration of outcome [3].

Surgery also creates a portal for introduction of infection in noncompound injuries. In these patients, the infection may be more indolent. Immunocompromised patients are at increased risk for infection. Patients who have diabetes or rheumatoid arthritis are at risk for greater infection complications, particularly if the disease is controlled poorly. Hematogenous spread of infection to the foot or ankle joints or bones is extremely rare, even in patients who have significant immune compromise (Fig. 2).

A history of rapid deterioration of a joint that otherwise should have remained functional should raise suspicion of infection. Wound drainage after the ini-

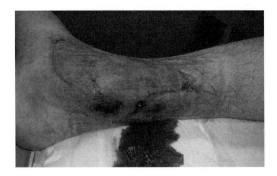

Fig. 2. Sinus tract indicative of infection despite free flap coverage of a reconstructed ankle fracture. The patient had poorly controlled rheumatoid arthritis as a risk factor for infection and wound necrosis. The patient declined ankle fusion; debridement was performed.

tial surgery, recurrent cellulitis, or sinus tract formation is highly suspicious for ongoing sepsis. Rapid loss of bone after the initial treatment also should raise concern.

Physical examination may support these findings. Swelling of the extremity and thickened subcutaneous tissues are suggestive of infection. During physical examination the surgeon should assess the integrity of the soft tissue envelope. Thickened and rigid skin may compromise exposure and closure. Multiple and tethered scars also may prevent appropriate exposure and cause wound edge necrosis. Transverse scars and scars over bone and tendon may be particularly problematic.

If there is an area of incomplete healing or granulation tissue, the area needs to be debrided to allow adequate visualization. After the area has been exposed, the tract can be examined. A sterile probe or Q-tip should be used. If the probe passes deep to the skin, and specifically probes to bone or hardware, a surgical debridement is likely the only method by which infection can be eradicated. Sinus tracts need to be excised and debrided. If a difficult closure is anticipated, a plastic surgical consult should be obtained. Tissue expansion or free flaps obtain the soft tissue coverage that is essential for infection eradication [4].

Preoperative investigations

Bloodwork

In patients with an appropriate history, thoughtful investigation should be performed. All at-risk patients should have a complete blood cell (CBC) count, erythrocyte sedimentation rate (ESR), and C-reactive protein (CRP) performed. A CBC count is unlikely to be abnormal in all but the most septic patients. ESR and CRP are the most sensitive and specific preoperative indicators of infection, particularly if both are abnormal [5]. A patient who has a fracture and abnormal blood results with no other cause (ie, other known source of infection or inflammatory systemic disease) should be assumed to have an infection within the fracture site or joint until proven otherwise.

Cultures

Preoperative determination of the organism is of benefit so that correct postoperative antibiotic treatment can be initiated. Patients should be off all antibiotics before culture or aspiration. Ideally, three cultures should be obtained to reduce the sampling error.

An aspiration of a deep abscess cavity, nonunion site, or joint can be performed under fluoroscopic control. Cultures should be sent for aerobic and anaerobic cultures, and at least three samples should be sent to avoid sampling error. On occasion, no cavity exists in which an aspiration can be performed. In this case, a tissue or bone biopsy of a suspicious area can be performed. This can be directed by fluoroscopic or CT control.

Superficial skin cultures are of no diagnostic or therapeutic benefit. Therefore, the surgeon should know from where previous specimens were obtained and ensure their validity.

Imaging

Serial radiographs should be reviewed to determine if a specific area of bone lysis has developed. Standing plain radiographs of the affected region of the foot or ankle should be obtained. In cases where significant loss of bone may be present, a CT scan allows more precise determination of bone loss. Defects may be cavitary or segmental. Cavitary defects may be filled with cancellous bone during reconstruction, whereas segmental defects require a segmental bone graft [6]. The CT scan also allows the surgeon to identify dead bone segments that act as foreign bodies and should be removed.

Aspiration

Aspiration of a joint may allow the surgeon to identify the organism involved. Local anesthetic injected into the joint allows the surgeon to confirm the origin of pain.

Culture of sinus tract

Skin cultures are of little use because they always are positive. Identification of resistant organisms (methicillin-resistant *Staphylococcus aureus* or vancomycin-resistant *Enterococcus*) may be the only beneficial finding of a skin culture. A needle should be inserted next to a sinus tract to aspirate the deep tissue rather than culture directly from the sinus tract.

MRI

MRI can be of use in determining the extent of infection within the bone marrow or soft tissues. MRI also can be used to assess a tendon sheath infection; however, it may be oversensitive for determining the extent of infection, and needs to be performed with a specific goal in mind.

Ultrasound

Ultrasound can be a quick and efficient way of assessing the extent of a soft tissue infection. An abscess cavity can be aspirated under ultrasound control and allows correct identification of the infecting organism. Ultrasound drainage of an abscess cavity and insertion of a pigtail catheter can be used as a temporary nonoperative measure in sicker patients.

Intraoperative management of an infected traumatized joint

The surgical goals can be divided into several specific steps:

Identification of the infecting organism
Infection eradication by complete debridement
Joint reconstruction or fusion
Soft tissue closure

All of these goals must be planned preoperatively, and must be completed intraoperatively. For example, infection eradication cannot be achieved without fusion of infected destroyed joints or adequate soft tissue coverage [7]. If the joint is viable, infection eradication and soft tissue coverage may suffice. Fusion cannot be achieved if infection eradication is incomplete or if soft tissue coverage is not achieved.

The infected posttraumatic joint also may fall in the following categories:

Known infection with pus and necrotic tissue
Known infection with skin coverage problems or a sinus tract
Known infection with good skin coverage and no pus
Joint appears infected during surgery
Joint diagnosed as infected after surgery

Intraoperative identification of infecting organism

A discussion with a microbiologist at your hospital will help to determine a watertight protocol for the correct diagnosis and treatment of infecting organisms. The authors' protocol involves taking at least three specimens, including bone or synovium. Tissue also should be sent for histology.

Three specimens are taken because false positives can occur between the operating room, sampling techniques, and plating out in the laboratory. False negatives also can occur depending on the site cultured, and the transport time and technique in the laboratory. Three specimens that are all positive with the same organism and same sensitivity allow a fairly robust diagnosis of infection. Similarly, three negative cultures (with the patient off antibiotics preoperatively) confirm a clean wound site.

Frozen sections can assist in the intraoperative diagnosis of infection. More than 5 or 10 white blood cells per high-power field are considered by different investigators to be the diagnostic for infected joint replacement. Similar standards can be used for infected hardware, soft tissue, or bone; however the pathologist needs to be comfortable with the technique, and the surgeon must sample infected tissue correctly. Inflamed tissue next to hardware may be the most appropriate tissue sample [8].

Gram stains have little diagnostic capability. The only time that the Gram stain is of intraoperative use is to confirm the presence of infection when a bacterium is seen. Otherwise a Gram stain has poor sensitivity and specificity [9].

Specimens should be marked correctly for aerobic and anaerobic culture, to differentiate the specimen as a surgical specimen, rather than as a routine skin culture. If the laboratory cannot identify the specimen correctly, the culture may be interpreted as normal skin commensals and no further identification or sensitivities provided. Alerting the laboratory to the specimens also is helpful. The operating room staff should call for a porter to ensure that the cultures are not left sitting for prolonged periods of time. Better still, the laboratory should be altered to receive an intraoperative specimen Specimens also should be sent for histopathology. The presence of inflammatory cells can help in the diagnosis of infection.

To ensure that no sample is discarded by the laboratory registration desk, the authors label all samples with a different site (eg, medial malleolus, lateral malleolus, and distal tibia for an ankle specimen). Often, laboratory reception desks are instructed to discard duplicate requests, which reduces the diagnostic ability for infection.

What is done with the information gained above the surgeon must decide. If there are more than five white blood cells per high-power field, an infection of some magnitude probably is present. There always is a delay between the taking, transportation, and analysis of the samples. While waiting, the debridement and exposure should be continued, with the operative plan being modified depending on the result of the frozen section. The surgeon may choose to defer definitive fixation, or may add a bead pouch or antibiotic pellets to the reconstruction.

Known infection with pus and necrotic tissue

If the patient has known infection with pus and necrotic tissue, the surgeon must have a dialog with the patient about reasonable goals with surgery. The patient is at significant risk for having a below-knee amputation if treatment fails.

If a rapid recovery is required, a below-knee amputation may be the primary treatment choice.

If the limb is to be salvaged the surgeon needs to articulate the goals, risks, and benefits of the surgery clearly [3]. The surgeon always should discuss the alternative of a below-knee amputation with the patient before initiating treatment.

If necrosis and pus are present the surgeon may elect to do a two-stage procedure: debriding the joint and removing all infected tissue, which is followed by a second-stage fusion. Antibiotic spacers may be required. The authors used to use this protocol, but found that with external fixation they could achieve the goals with a single-stage procedure [10].

Technique of single-stage salvage of infected joint

After appropriate preparation and draping, the joint is exposed using extensile exposures that accommodate any previous incisions. A complete debridement is performed; all hardware (including broken screws) and necrotic bone and tissue are removed.

The remaining bone stock is assessed by using preoperative CT scanning. The joint is prepared for fusion by preparing congruent joint surfaces in the neutral position. Bone graft may be required for cavitary defects—an autologous graft is preferable to an allograft—and all being used after careful consideration of infection risk. In this environment large segmental grafts should not be used; the authors have used OsteoSet beads (Wright Medical, Memphis, Tennessee) with tobramycin. If bone graft is necessary, another option is to use cancellous graft mixed with tobramycin powder. The elution of the antibiotic is excellent, and does not interfere in any way with graft incorporation. In some cases saw cuts may be used to create opposing bone ends, at the cost of limb length.

In the face of significant pus or necrosis, internal fixation should be avoided; the authors apply an external fixator. First, the opposing joint surfaces should be held reduced with a percutaneous wire or pin that is removed after application of an external fixator. OsteoSet beads with tobramycin, vancomycin, or both antibiotics are placed around the joint margins. The wounds are closed; if tight, a vacuum dressing is applied [11].

An external fixator is applied. For ankle fusions, half-pin fixation is used on the tibia, with fixation achieved on both sides of the foot by way of fine wire fixation or through-and-through pin fixation. The joint is compressed, and the temporary fixation wire is removed. If a temporary fixation wire is not used, the OsteoSet beads will fall between the bone ends and prevent bone apposition. The wound should be closed before application of the fixator because the entry points of the pins through the skin cannot be judged with the wounds open, and closure of the wounds is much harder when working around the external fixator (Fig. 3).

Postoperative antibiotics are administered for 6 weeks; the drugs of choice are determined by the intraoperative culture results. The external fixator is removed at 3 to 4 months after surgery, and the patient immobilized in a cast if required.

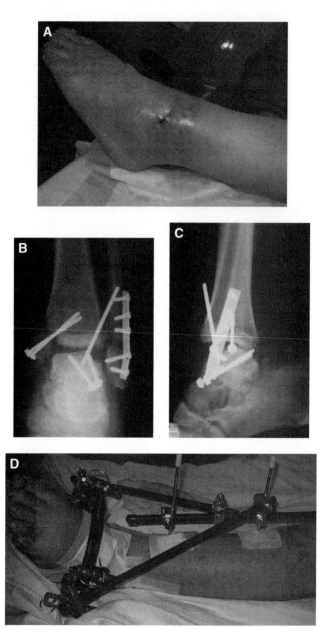

Fig. 3. (*A*) A preoperative clinical photograph of a patient who had a draining sinus after open reduction and internal fixation of a compound ankle fracture 8 months earlier. The foot is fixed in equinus. Plain radiographs (*B, C*) and clinical photograph (*D*) of the same patient after single-stage debridement, insertion of antibiotic beads, and application of an external fixator. (*E, F*) Final views after removal of the external fixator showing a plantar grade foot and solid tibiotalar fusion.

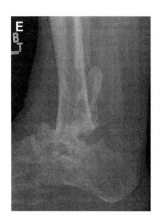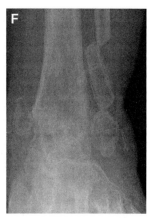

Fig. 3 (*continued*).

Known infection with minimal bone involvement, no pus, and no sinus tract

In some cases after trauma the joint becomes arthritic rapidly, with abnormal ESRs and CRPs, and possibly, a positive culture. In these cases a joint infection may be known or strongly suspected. A weak pathogen may be present within the joint.

A CT scan should be performed before surgical treatment to assess bone stock. Stabilization with internal fixation can be performed; however, complete removal of all old hardware, including broken screws, is required because glycocalyx-forming organisms can cause treatment failure.

After hardware removal and joint surface preparation, stable internal fixation is required. OsteoSet beads with vancomycin or tobramycin may be placed around the fusion site. Stable fixation must be achieved because the joint can be considered to act like an infected nonunion. Articles about fractures and animal models showed that infection eradication can be achieved more easily with stable fixation than with minimal or no internal fixation. Postoperative antibiotic coverage is directed by culture results. A standard protocol is used postoperatively (Fig. 4).

Known infection with soft tissue coverage problems

Adequate soft tissue coverage is a prerequisite for infection eradication. Because most infecting organisms are skin commensals an appropriate skin barrier is required between the joint and the outside. The additional circulation of an appropriate skin flap or free flap assists in bone healing and infection eradication. The joint should be managed as outlined above for infection. Any joint with poor soft tissue coverage should be assumed to be infected until culture results are returned.

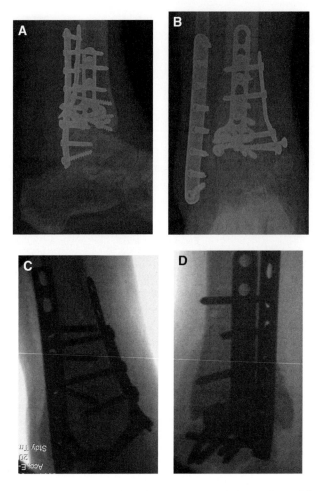

Fig. 4. 85-year-old independent patient who underwent an open reduction and internal fixation (ORIF) of a distal tibia fracture 1 year before presentation. (*A–B*) She had been admitted on two or three occasions for cellulitis and swelling of the ankle. Her ESR at presentation was 70. She had delayed wound healing after the ORIF. Intraoperative views. (*C–D*) She had poor bone stock and the fractures were ununited. The bone was soft and fragmented with screw insertion. There was no pus present, and intraoperative cultures confirmed infection. She was treated with antibiotics for 6 weeks.

Patients who have suspected intraoperative infection not suspected preoperatively

In patients who have a joint that looks suspicious for infection intraoperatively, cultures are taken using the aforementioned guidelines. An immediate post-operative ESR or CRP should be obtained to assist in the diagnosis. The joint should be fused or stabilized as determined by the preoperative plan, and OsteoSet beads with tobramycin may be used instead of bone graft.

The patient is kept on an empiric choice of antibiotics (cephalexin or van-comycin with ciprofloxacin) until the culture results return. The patient may be switched to an oral protocol if the organism is sensitive to an oral agent [12]. If all investigations come back negative, the patient can be treated without any further antibiotic coverage.

Patients with a postoperative diagnosis of infection

On occasion, a patient has a fusion or osteotomy performed, which is followed by a postoperative diagnosis of infection based on an intraoperative culture. In these cases the cultures should be reviewed with the microbiologist to determine

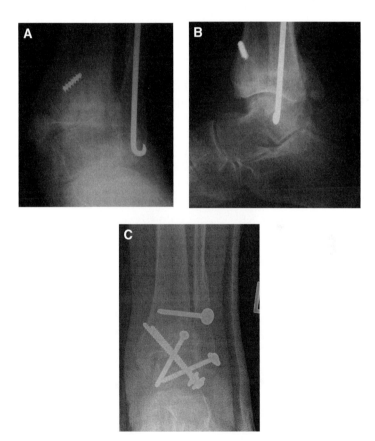

Fig. 5. (*A–C*) A woman who had early collapse after an open reduction and internal fixation of an ankle fracture and partial hardware removal. After surgery, drainage occurred and a preoperative aspiration was positive for infection (Corynebacterium). Her ESR (60 mm in first hour) and CRP (16 mg/L) were abnormal. Surgical treatment included a single-stage debridement and ankle fusion using OsteoSet beads, followed by a 6-week course of antibiotics. All old hardware was removed. Postoperative views. A solid ankle fusion was achieved with insertion of antibiotic pellets loaded with tobramycin. The ESR was 26 at 3 months after surgery and the fusion was healed.

if the specimen is a contaminant. If infection is suspected after this discussion the patient should be treated with the appropriate antibiotic regime. Any hardware that was not removed during the procedure may need to be removed to ensure successful eradication of infection (Fig. 5).

Joint salvage versus fusion versus replacement in the face of infection

The diagnosis of infection usually means that the joint concerned has lost articular cartilage; therefore, in most cases it cannot be salvaged by osteotomy or debridement. In questionable cases, assessment of the joint surface can be performed by arthroscopy or MRI examination.

On occasion, a patient requests an ankle joint replacement for reconstruction of an infected, traumatized ankle. This can be performed only by a two-stage procedure that is similar to those outlined for infected total joint replacement [13,14]. In the first stage the ankle is debrided and a spacer placed, or a fusion is performed.

If a spacer is placed, the patient should have a 6-week course of antibiotics, which is followed by 6 weeks of observation to allow the soft tissue envelope to settle. The cuts that are required for the joint replacement can be performed at the first stage before spacer placement. Repeat ESR and CRP should show a reduction if infection has been eradicated.

Repeat aspiration around the spacer should show infection eradication. With this protocol, as used for infected hip and knee joint replacements, an infection eradication rate of 90% should be possible if good skin coverage can be achieved.

References

[1] Christiano RA, Bos KE. Management of chronic osteomyelitis of the lower extremity. Neth J Surg 1988;40(3):76–9.

[2] Dubey L, Krasinski K, Hernanz-Schulman M. Osteomyelitis secondary to trauma or infected contiguous soft tissue. Pediatr Infect Dis J 1988;7(1):26–34.

[3] Hulscher JB, te Velde EA, Schuurman AH, et al. Arthrodesis after osteosynthesis and infection of the ankle joint. Injury 2001;32(2):145–52.

[4] Baumeister S, Germann G. Soft tissue coverage of the extremely traumatized foot and ankle. Foot Ankle Clin 2001;6(4):867–903.

[5] Spangehl MJ, Younger AS, Masri BA, et al. Diagnosis of infection following total hip arthroplasty. Instr Course Lect 1998;47:285–95.

[6] Paprosky WG, Perona PG, Lawrence JM. Acetabular defect classification and surgical reconstruction in revision arthroplasty. A 6-year follow-up evaluation. J Arthroplasty 1994; 9(1):33–44.

[7] Worlock P, Slack R, Harvey L, et al. The prevention of infection in open fractures: an experimental study of the effect of fracture stability. Injury 1994;25(1):31–8.

[8] Della Valle CJ, Bogner E, Desai P, et al. Analysis of frozen sections of intraoperative specimens obtained at the time of reoperation after hip or knee resection arthroplasty for the treatment of infection. J Bone Joint Surg Am 1999;81(5):684–9.

[9] Della Valle CJ, Scher DM, Kim YH, et al. The role of intraoperative Gram stain in revision total joint arthroplasty. J Arthroplasty 1999;14(4):500–4.

[10] Lortat-Jacob A, Beaufils P, Coignard S, et al. [Tibiotarsal arthrodesis in a septic milieu]. Rev Chir Orthop Reparatrice Appar Mot 1984;70(6):449–56.

[11] Mullner T, Mrkonjic L, Kwasny O, et al. The use of negative pressure to promote the healing of tissue defects: a clinical trial using the vacuum sealing technique. Br J Plast Surg 1997; 50(3):194–9.

[12] Swiontkowski MF, Hanel DP, Vedder NB, et al. A comparison of short- and long-term intravenous antibiotic therapy in the postoperative management of adult osteomyelitis. J Bone Joint Surg Br 1999;81(6):1046–50.

[13] Younger AS, Duncan CP, Masri BA. Treatment of infection associated with segmental bone loss in the proximal part of the femur in two stages with use of an antibiotic-loaded interval prosthesis. J Bone Joint Surg Am 1998;80(1):60–9.

[14] Younger AS, Duncan CP, Masri BA, et al. The outcome of two-stage arthroplasty using a custom-made interval spacer to treat the infected hip. J Arthroplasty 1997;12(6):615–23.

ELSEVIER
SAUNDERS

Foot Ankle Clin N Am
11 (2006) 217–235

FOOT AND
ANKLE CLINICS

Soft Tissue Coverage for Posttraumatic Reconstruction

Alastair S.E. Younger, MB, ChB, MSc, ChM, FRCSC[a,b,]*, Tom Goetz, MD[a]

[a]*Department of Orthopaedics, The University of British Columbia, 401-1160 Burrard Street, Vancouver, British Columbia V6Z 2E8, Canada*
[b]*British Columbia's Foot and Ankle Clinic, Providence Health Care, Vancouver, British Columbia, Canada*

Assessment of the soft tissue envelope around the foot and ankle is essential before undertaking posttraumatic reconstruction. The original injury and treatment may leave a soft tissue envelope that will not tolerate a reconstructive procedure. Careful assessment of the soft tissue envelope and appropriate planning of the skin incision may avoid or identify the need for a soft tissue reconstructive procedure. Preoperative identification of the need for soft tissue reconstruction provides an immediate, stable soft tissue envelope in the postoperative period, allows earlier rehabilitation, and decreases the risk for catastrophic wound infection [1].

Occasionally, and often despite careful planning, postoperative wound breakdown may occur. Early wound care and the use of new wound care modalities, such as vacuum-assisted wound closure (VAC; KCI, San Antonio, Texas), may allow wound healing without the need for difficult and costly soft tissue procedures [2]. Failing this, early surgical soft tissue coverage should be undertaken to improve outcome [1].

Many wounds can be managed by dressings alone. If the wound is small and is not associated with deep infection of avascular tissue or implants, it will heal. Many dressings have been advocated, but few have any form of scientific evidence as to their effect. Platelet-derived growth factor gels (Regranex, Johnson

* Corresponding author. 401-1160 Burrard Street, Vancouver, British Columbia V6Z 2E8, Canada.
E-mail address: asyounger@shaw.ca (A.S.E. Younger).

1083-7515/06/$ – see front matter © 2006 Elsevier Inc. All rights reserved.
doi:10.1016/j.fcl.2005.12.009
foot.theclinics.com

& Johnson, Somerville, New Jersey), skin allograft (Dermagraft, Smith & Nephew, Inc., La Jolla, California) and graft jacket (Wright Medical, Arlington, Tennessee), hyperbaric oxygen [3], and collagen dressings (Promagran, Johnson & Johnson) are agents that have been promoted to stimulate wound healing.

A free flap may be required before reconstruction. In other circumstances, a free flap may be required after reconstruction. The choice of free flap, with respect to donor site and depth (fascial, fascial and muscle, or osteocutaneous) depends on the defect that needs to be filled. In all cases, the earlier that the soft tissue compromise is recognized and treated, the faster the patient will rehabilitate and the better the prognosis will be.

Assessing the risk for soft tissue complications

Preoperative assessment

Before undertaking any posttraumatic reconstruction of the ankle, the surgeon should undertake a preoperative assessment. An assessment of the soft tissue envelope allows the surgeon to evaluate the potential for soft tissue healing complications. This is pertinent in posttraumatic reconstruction because of the likelihood of deformity and scarring from the trauma's previous surgical repair. Careful surgical planning can avoid the need for complex soft tissue reconstructive procedures, and minimize the chance of wound breakdown. These may lead to deep infection or a delay in mobilization, both of which can lead to amputation. Identification of the need for soft tissue reconstruction before surgery allows a coordinated multidisciplinary approach and decreases the risks for catastrophic failure. Soft tissue reconstruction that is performed at the time of the index reconstructive procedure is preferable to postoperative wound breakdown. Surgeon experience is most valuable in determining soft tissue coverage needs. Certain principles are described that assist the surgeon in avoiding pitfalls.

Assessment is divided into patient factors, extremity factors, and local wound factors. These factors are evaluated through history, physical examination, and pertinent investigations. This allows the determination of feasibility and risk for a reconstructive procedure and the identification of risk factors and contraindications.

Patient factors

A thorough medical history identifies conditions that may affect wound healing. The patient must be healthy enough to withstand the surgical procedure and the necessary rehabilitation. Cardiac, respiratory, and renal disease must be evaluated by subspecialty consultation, and need to be optimized or corrected before surgery. Coagulopathies must be corrected. Factors that affect wound healing need to be considered.

Diabetes causes wound-healing problems, increased infection rates, renal disease, increased risk for comorbid disease, and—through its effect on small vessels—peripheral neuropathy and small vessel disease. Long-standing and poorly controlled diabetes increases these risks. Hemoglobin A1c (HbA1c) can evaluate diabetic control. Severe diabetes merits careful vascular assessment. Local tissue transfer with pedicle flaps is often compromised and micro ascular anastomosis with free flaps becomes technically challenging.

A history of smoking affects wound healing adversely. A social history may reveal an inability to understand the objectives, risks, and benefits of the reconstructive procedure, or an inability to comply with the postoperative protocol. A history of intravenous (IV) drug abuse or significant psychiatric disease may be a contraindication for surgery.

Adequate patient resources will be required for postoperative care, splinting/bracing, and mobility devices.

Extremity factors

Arterial peripheral vascular disease is evident with a history of dependent rubor, claudication, and atrophic shiny skin. Evidence of arterial insufficiency or absence of peripheral pulses merits vascular assessment. Venous insufficiency is evidenced by chronic edema and discoloration of the extremity. There may be a history of deep venous thrombosis, varicose veins, or vein stripping.

Loss of sensation or neuropathy also may compromise the outcome of a soft tissue reconstruction.

Local wound factors

The reconstructive procedure needs to take into account previous trauma to the foot and ankle. A significant deformity correction may be planned that may leave a soft tissue deficit that requires soft tissue coverage. The existing soft tissue cover may be inadequate. Severe scarring or previous split-thickness skin grafting will not tolerate flap elevation well. Tendon transfers cannot be passed through such poor skin. Skin mobility can be assessed to determine compliance, and the ability to rotate local random flaps. Skin flaps cannot be elevated in region of skin grafting. Incisions through these zones are possible if they are elevated full thickness, down to bone.

Previous scars need to be considered when planning skin incisions. Ideally, the previous scar should be used. Incisions that are placed parallel to or that cross scars at acute angles can cause tissue necrosis. Open wounds or ulcers may be present. Reconstruction must be planned to allow healing or coverage.

Technical investigations

With clinical evidence of arterial insufficiency, Doppler pressures should be measured. Pressures that are less than 50 mm Hg indicate arterial compromise

[4]. An ankle–brachial index of less than 0.8 indicates arterial obstruction. An occlusive pressure measurement is not reliable in diabetic patients [5].

Specific local and regional flaps can be evaluated by a Doppler probe to assess their blood supply. The dorsalis pedis or medial plantar flap may require such an assessment.

In diabetics the peroneal artery often is spared from vascular disease, which allows the use of local flaps (eg, sural flap). Any local flap that requires posterior tibialis artery patency is not possible with an absent posterior tibialis pulse unless bypass grafting is performed first.

Arteriography is indicated if a free flap is contemplated in an extremity with significant past trauma or multiple surgeries, or when pulses cannot be palpated easily.

Making the decision about the need for coverage

A vascular surgeon consultation is required in any case where there is insufficient blood flow to allow for wound healing. If significant peripheral arterial disease is present with arterial occlusion and there is a need for a free flap, a vascular procedure may be performed before the reconstruction to provide inflow for a free flap. Generally, 4 weeks are required before the risk for graft thrombosis is minimized. An alternative is to have a vascular surgeon create an arteriovenous shunt. This brings a loop of vein graft to the region of the reconstruction. The soft tissue surgeon may then cut the loop to provide arterial inflow and venous outflow.

Prevention of wound complications

Many wound complications that are seen in reconstruction can be traced back to poor decisions that were made at the time of the initial surgery. Longitudinal incisions that lend themselves to extensile exposures should be used. Skin bridges must be planned, and excessive subcutaneous dissection must be avoided. Ideally, incisions should be placed over viable muscle, rather than over tendons or bones (Fig. 1).

For a distal tibial fracture, a longitudinal anterior incision allows excellent exposure to the joint line and is extensile. The curvilinear anterior incision is hard to use because the saphenous nerve and the anterior tendons prevent easy exposure. The wound is not extensile for late reconstruction. A longitudinal anterior lateral incision allows late reconstruction if the incision is not curved.

The initial surgery should be planned at a time when the soft tissue envelope will tolerate surgery. Incisions should avoid fracture blisters [6]. Blood-filled fracture blisters may be more problematic than serum-filled blisters. The wrinkle test (when swelling has diminished to the point that the skin will wrinkle) is used to determine when surgery can be performed safely [7].

In some cases, wounds cannot be closed easily at the time of initial surgery. The use of a VAC dressing or delayed primary closure may be appropriate [8]. Multiple small incisions (pie crusting) may allow the skin to be closed (Fig. 2). The small relaxing incisions will heal by secondary re-epithelization, much like a skin graft. The use of a skin graft over a wound is preferable to a tight

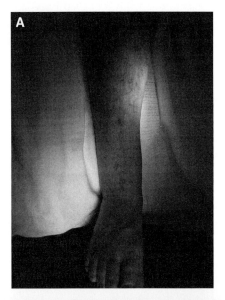

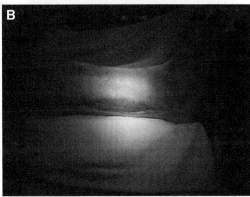

Fig. 1. Longitudinal incisions used for an open reduction of a tibia plafond associated with a compartment syndrome. The initial management included a compartment release and external fixation. All incisions were longitudinal and over muscle. This allowed a subsequent posterior medial approach to the posterior compartment without compromise of the older style hockey stick incision. (*A*) Anterior longitudinal incision. (*B*) Lateral incision. (*C*) Later posterior medial approach. (*D*) Traditional anterior approach to a distal tibial fracture that does not allow extensile exposure for late reconstruction as demonstrated in (*C*).

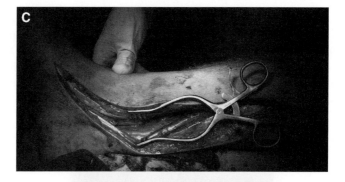

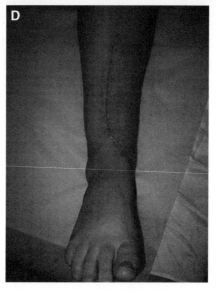

Fig. 1 (*continued*).

closure and skin necrosis. This may act as a temporary dressing that assists in salvaging all available tissue until definitive skin coverage, or it may provide definitive closure.

Achilles tendon incisions should be kept off the midline (Fig. 3).

In most cases, late reconstruction allows the surgeon to set the stage for a successful procedure. Various systemic factors can be addressed during the preoperative work-up. Poorly controlled diabetes has a significant effect on wound healing. An HbA1c of greater than 8% is associated with poor wound healing of diabetic ulcers [9,10]. Achieving an HbA1c level that is less than this before surgery may prevent wound complications. Maintaining good post-operative glucose control (< 10 mmol/L or < 180 mg/dL) also reduces the rate of wound infections.

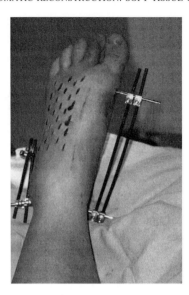

Fig. 2. Pie crusting at the time of injury allows better soft tissue healing. A similar technique can be used at late reconstruction to detension a wound closure. (Courtesy of Richard DiGiovanni, MD, *From* Browner B, Trafton P, Green N, et al, editors. Skeletal trauma. 3rd edition. Philadelphia: WB Saunders; 2003, with permission.)

Patients who have systemic rheumatoid diseases may have a history of vasculitis. Consultation with a rheumatologist preoperatively allows for optimization of medical treatment that may prevent postoperative wound necrosis. Prolonged treatment with prednisone can cause poor wound healing and vascular compromise (Fig. 4).

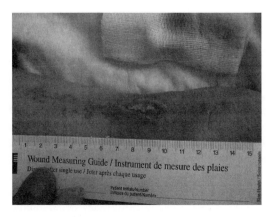

Fig. 3. Medial incision line for Achilles tendon repair. In the case of wound necrosis, the medial placement may allow for conservative treatment if a posterior incision results in exposure and infection of the tendon.

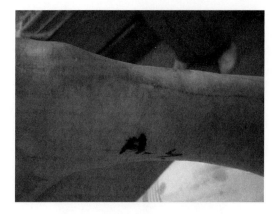

Fig. 4. This patient, who had systemic lupus erythematosus and was on long-term prednisone treatment, had an Achilles tendon rupture that was missed. The wound broke down at late reconstruction, and a sinus developed 4 weeks after surgery. Two debridements and removal of all stitch material effected a cure. This illustrates the risk for operations on the Achilles tendon for patients who have systemic disease and trauma.

All patients must have palpable pulses before reconstruction. If one pulse is missing, vascular assessment is appropriate. Pulses may be missing because of congenital variations, vessel damage from previous surgery or injury, or occlusive arterial disease. Wound necrosis can be predicted in these cases, and may change the incisions that are used.

Patients with a history of delayed wound healing should have a more detailed vascular examination. If all pulses are not palpable, investigation should include Doppler mapping of the vessels, plus determination of ankle–brachial indices [7,11]. Vascular surgical consultation should be performed. Venous insufficiency also should be recognized and treated, if present. Poor nutrition and low hemoglobin count also should be treated.

Smoking and vasoconstrictive drugs, such as cocaine, have a major effect on wound healing [9,12]. Specific enquiry about drug abuse, smoking, and the cessation of smoking is required. The authors avoid operating on anyone who uses cocaine or related drugs, or who smokes.

In the operating room, tourniquet times should be kept to a minimum. Appropriate hemostasis should be obtained before wound closure. Incisions should be planned carefully. Ideally, wounds that had healing problems previously should be avoided (Fig. 5). If wound-healing issues are anticipated, a preoperative plastic surgical consult may be appropriate.

On occasion, arthroscopic surgery may be used to avoid wound complications. Arthroscopic-assisted ankle or subtalar fusion may be an alternative for patients who have a history of wound healing problems (Fig. 6).

Extensive soft tissue dissection should be avoided. A new longitudinal incision should be used while taking into account the angiosomes of the foot. If a

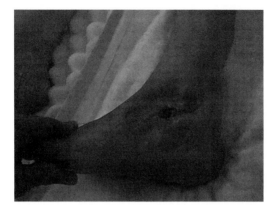

Fig. 5. Posttraumatic calcaneocuboid joint arthritis. The patient had an old oblique approach to the sinus tarsi from a subtalar fusion. The new incision broke down, with exposure to the plate. The wound was managed successfully by dressing with Iodosorb and leaving the plate in place until the joint fused. The plate was removed, and the wound closed successfully.

transverse incision has been used before, the new incision should cross the old incision at 90° to reduce the chance of wound necrosis.

Deep dissection should be performed carefully. Prolonged use of self-retaining retractors should be avoided. Sharp dissection damages the least number of cells in each layer. Hemostasis should be obtained during disection. Larger incisions without the use of excessive retraction are preferable to small incisions with retraction.

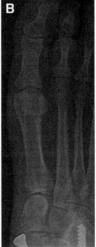

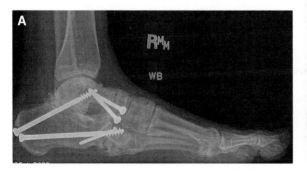

Fig. 6. Patient who had posttraumatic arthritis many years after a navicular fracture and skin loss over the lateral border of the foot with a healed skin graft and friable skin. The fusions of the subtalar and calcaneocuboid joints were performed arthroscopically with percutaneous screw fixation. This avoided lateral wound breakdown. Lateral (A) and anteroposterior (B) radiographs.

The tourniquet should be deflated before closure and hemostasis should be obtained. Wounds should be closed in layers without excessive suture material. Drains may assist in preventing hematoma formation. Skin closure should not be tight. Staples require more skin to close than do interrupted or continuous nylon; therefore, staples should be avoided if several incisions are present or if the wound closure is tight. An absorbable subcuticular stitch may cause an excessive soft tissue reaction that causes the wound to open; therefore, it should be avoided.

If an incision has one side that is at risk for necrosis, an Algower suture can be used. By being subcutaneous on one side, the wound edge blood supply is not compromised by the presence of a suture. An interrupted mattress suture may prevent wound problems in an at-risk wound.

Dressings should be loose and allow for absorption of blood. Tensor (Ace) bandages are wrapped loosely because they can cause excessive tension. Cast

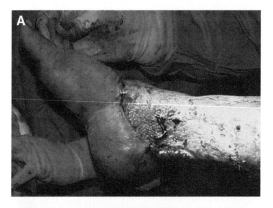

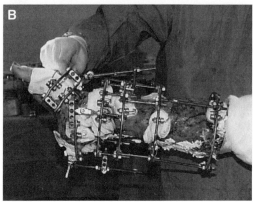

Fig. 7. (A) Patient who had a tibial fracture and an equinus contracture after a crush injury from a bus wheel. (B) An external fixator allowed access to extensive skin grafts for dressings and gradual correction of the equinus deformity. The authors often use an external fixator to hold correction in patients who have free flaps or soft tissue injuries and who cannot be casted.

material should be well padded and kept away from incision lines. Patients who have at-risk wounds should be admitted to the hospital for elevation of the limb. After discharge, instructions are given for continued elevation until wound review at 1 to 2 weeks.

On occasion, the use of external fixation can be used for patients who have poor soft tissue envelopes (Fig. 7).

Management of wound problems

Despite taking care with incisions and treatment, surgeons find themselves troubled by wound complications. Most of these can be managed without further surgical treatment.

Minor wound problems

Minor subcutaneous stitch abscesses and wound breakdown can be treated by debridement, removal of any foreign material, and polysporin application by the patient with a single-layer dressing. These wounds should be less than 5 mm wide, have a granulating base with no drainage and no exposed bone or tendon, and have a closed subcutaneous layer. The value of hyperbaric oxygen is debatable as a wound healing adjunct [13].

A stable black eschar can be watched with iodine painted around the wound edge. Debridement should be delayed if drainage is minimal, because debridement may remove underlying viable epithelial cells. The eschar eventually separates to reveal underlying new skin or granulation tissue.

Dressings

Modern wound dressings that need to be changed three times a week are preferable to more traditional daily dressings if assistance from home care is required.

Cadexomer iodine (Iodosorb; Smith & Nephew) is a starch gel with impregnated iodine. The serum in the wound gradually allows the iodine to be released into the wound; this prevents excessive bacterial colonization and is nontoxic to the surrounding tissues. Wounds that are up to 5 to 6 cm in length with deep communication to bone or tendon can be treated with Iodosorb dressings as a temporary measure, although these wounds can also heal completely with this type of dressing. Studies showed that these dressings are more cost effective, and are as efficient as daily wet to dry dressings [14]. Debridement of the wound should be performed first [15].

Acticoat (Smith & Nephew) is a nanocrystalline silver-based dressing that allows a gradual release of silver into the wound. The silver acts as a bactericidal agent, and controls methicillin-resistant *Staphylococcus aureus*. Dressings are changed two to three times weekly. The authors prefer to use the silver dressing for shallow wounds with less exudate, and Iodosorb for deeper wounds.

Caustic agents, such as Dakin's solution, should be avoided because they may cause significant tissue necrosis and prevent wound healing.

Debridement of wounds is better performed by sharp dissection when indicated in the clinic. Chemical agents may not prevent bacterial colonization and may cause skin maceration. After sharp debridement, appropriate dressings can be placed on the wound base.

Sugar and honey prevent bacterial colonization in a similar way by osmotic pressure. Daily dressings are required and can be performed by the compliant patient.

Vacuum-assisted closure dressings

VAC using negative pressure wound therapy can be used for wounds that are hard to close at the time of the initial surgery, or for infected wounds that require drainage [2,16]. Negative pressure is applied to the wound by way of a polypropylene sponge. The treatment allows granulation tissue to form, probably by bringing serum into the wound [17]. The negative pressure may assist in bringing the wound edges together, particularly in mobile posttraumatic wounds [18]. A randomized prospective study showed some benefit in wound healing [8]. Edema and bacterial counts within the wound also may be reduced by the treatment. VAC dressings have been used in the authors' clinic more for inpatient care and for early wound complications, although outpatient treatment can be provided.

A VAC dressing can be used in combination with a skin graft or skin graft substitute, such as graft jacket or dermagraft [19,20]. The use of a skin graft may accelerate the wound closure compared with using a VAC dressing alone.

Slow-healing granulating wounds

Occasionally, a granulating wound can be slow to heal. The surgeon should recheck the blood supply to the extremity, and confirm the presence of all major pulses using a Doppler probe if necessary. If any deficit exists, vascular surgical consultation and arterial imaging is appropriate. If other systemic factors have been addressed (eg, smoking, diet, diabetic control), several options exist for the further treatment of these wounds.

Autologous platelet-rich plasma can stimulate wound healing [21,22]. The authors have used autologous platelet concentrate with success in stimulating new granulation and epithelialization in a static wound; however, no formal study has been performed to support the technique.

Hyperbaric oxygen also has been advocated as a treatment for static wounds. The patient must be medically fit for the dive. The higher oxygen content under pressure is believed to assist in wound oxygenation and healing [23]. Studies about its value are inconclusive.

Major wound problems

In cases in which the wound is not predicted to heal, or if deep tissues may be compromised by prolonged dressings, a free flap may be indicated. Exposed bone needs to be covered if fracture healing or infection eradication is to be achieved. A free flap results in better local blood flow than does a skin graft or granulation tissue. An early free flap in cases that are not predicted to heal by wound size or exposed structures has better results than does expectant treatment followed by a late flap.

Several choices exist for tissue coverage. Traditionally, a tube pedicle graft was used to cover large lesions. Occasionally, a tube pedicle graft may be used if no other alternative exists (eg, patients who have reasonable capillary refill but no vessel large enough to feed a free flap) [24]. Vascular bypass surgery may be required before reconstruction is performed, because vascular compromise may be one of the causes of failed soft tissue coverage after trauma.

Local muscle flaps may be used for coverage; however these may be associated with significant donor site morbidity, and therefore, a free flap may be preferable [25]. The free flap may contain skin, fascia, muscle or bone, and feeding vessels. The choice of flap depends on the defect that needs to be filled [26]. Specific issues for free flaps in the foot include the need for shear resistance of plantar flaps, the effect of an insensate flap in a weight-bearing area, and the ability of the flap to adhere to the deep tissues [27]. Partial sensation can be restored to the flap if required [28].

The radial forearm is a common donor site for a fasciocutaneous flap because the donor site is remote, and a long vessel harvest can be achieved which allows anastomosis to the vessel distant to damaged tissue [29]. Innervation can be performed for this flap. The free scapular flap can be used for larger defects, although in larger patients the flap may be too thick to place in the foot easily.

Muscle flaps contain muscle, fascia, skin, and the vascular pedicle. Donor muscles include the gracilis, rectus abdominis, serratus, and latissimus dorsi. These flaps may have significant donor site morbidity. The muscle will bulk out a larger recipient site defect.

Osteocutaneous flaps contain bone, muscle, skin, and a vascular pedicle. Donor sites include the lateral arm and the radial forearm with a portion of the humerus or radius, respectively. A stress fracture may occur in the remaining donor bone; this is a particular risk for radial donor sites.

Options for soft tissue reconstruction

After the decision has been made that soft tissue coverage is required, the optimal coverage solution must be selected. Often, less surgery results in a better outcome. The simplest technique that meets the criteria for adequate coverage is the best technique. For example, if skin graft can be used for coverage, then it is the technique that should be used.

The location of the lesion determines the coverage that is required. The foot is divided into weight-bearing and nonweight-bearing regions. The weight-bearing areas are subdivided into the forefoot and the heel. The nonweight-bearing areas are divided into the ankle, the dorsum of the foot, and the instep.

Size of lesion

Wounds that are smaller than 4 to 5 cm^2 can be considered for local flap coverage. Larger lesions are treated best with free flaps. The depth of the wound and exposed structures affect the wound coverage options. Exposed tendon without paratenon and bone cannot be covered by skin graft, because the vascularity is inadequate to allow inosculation. Deeper wounds require bulk in tissue coverage; often, muscle flaps are best.

If the skin is scarred severely or is poorly mobile, indurated, or dysvascular it is not suitable for tissue shifts and local skin flaps. Poor vascularity of the foot and ankle suggests that local wound coverage will be inadequate. Free flaps will be more suitable, and bring healthy well-vascularized tissue to the wound [30].

Soft tissue coverage can be performed successfully on weight-bearing areas. Because of high contact and shear forces and insensitivity of the flaps there is a high rate of ulceration and hyperkeratosis. Sensation recovery is variable; some investigators suggested that there was no difference between reinnervated and insensate flaps, whereas others found good sensory recovery in innervated flaps. Deep sensation is present almost immediately and is likely from deeper structures [31].

The gold standard for soft tissue coverage in weight-bearing areas is a muscle flap that is covered by split-thickness skin graft, although other investigators favor fasciocutaneous flaps [26].

Skin grafting can be partial or full thickness. Skin grafting requires a clean, well-vascularized wound base. A skin graft will not take if there is infection and avascular or dysvascular tissue (eg, bone, tendon).

Anything that prevents inosculation to the skin graft from underlying tissue during the 3-to 5-day period that is required for in-growth of blood vessels will interfere with graft incorporation. During this period the graft survives by inosculation, or the transfer of nutrients from serum exudates. Increasing the thickness of the graft improves cosmoses and produces more durable coverage, but there is a decreased rate of take.

The authors prefer to use a split-thickness skin graft that is 18 thousands of an inch thickness. Pie crust is preferable to meshing for improved cosmoses. Pie crusting allows for drainage of blood to discourage hecatomb formation. It is helpful to place a bolster over the graft to ensure even pressure, and to decrease the risk for shear that is caused by loose dressings. It is the authors' practice to staple the edges of the graft and to cover it with wax-impregnated material. Normal saline–soaked gauze is applied; this is covered by a large, wax-impregnated dressing that is stapled down to apply pressure to the gauze bolster and the underlying skin graft. The bolster is left in place for 5 days, and the foot is kept elevated during this time. Dangling can begin after this time; continuous dependency is allowed at 2 weeks, and weight bearing on skin graft is allowed at 6 weeks.

Local tissue flaps

Local flaps allow for shorter operating time under potential regional anesthesia with lower preoperative risks. Local flaps replace tissue with like tissue, and there is no distant donor site morbidity. Local flaps have disadvantages, including local donor defect morbidity, limitation of the size of defect that can be covered, and sacrifice of a local artery. Local flap availability may be limited in the severely traumatized, dysvascular, and scarred limb.

Random pattern flaps do not rely on a vascular pedicle. Examples include Z-plasties, V-Y plasties, rotation plasties, and advancement and transposition flaps; all can provide coverage of small defects. The shifted tissue must have some compliance and normal vascularity. An example is the heel pad rotation flap for coverage of small heel defects [32]. Skin graft is required in the defect.

Wounds on the anterior ankle with small areas of breakdown can be treated with careful undermining and wound advancement.

Pedicled flaps are based on a known vascular pedicle [33]. The blood supply in the base of the pedicle should not have been damaged previously. Pedicled flaps can be local or regional.

A reverse neurofasciocutaneous flap can be used for soft tissue coverage of the lower leg. Flaps that are based on the cutaneous nerve distribution are well described [34,35]. They are reversed pedicled flaps that are supplied by the vascular network of the sensitive superficial nerves in the leg. Examples are the saphenous and the sural and lateral supramalleolar neurofasciocutaneous flaps.

The sural flap is pedicled on the neurovascular bundle that runs with the sural nerve. The maximum size is 10 cm × 13 cm; the pivot point is 5 cm proximal to the lateral malleolus. The flap is prone to venous congestion; in high-risk patients who have diabetes mellitus or peripheral vascular disease the complication rate can be as high as 25% [26].

The extensor digitorum brevis flap is based on the lateral tarsal artery. It is 4.5 cm × 6 cm in size and be mobilized to cover the ankle area [36]. It requires sacrifice of the anterior tibial artery.

The dorsalis pedis flap can be used as a local or free flap. It provides thin, pliable skin and can cover defects over the medial and lateral malleoli. It requires sacrifice of the dorsalis pedis artery and loss of superficial peroneal nerve sensation, and has an undesirable donor defect.

Free flaps

The advantages of free flaps are that they can cover large areas, allow selection of a variety of tissue types, and bring well-vascularized, undamaged tissue to

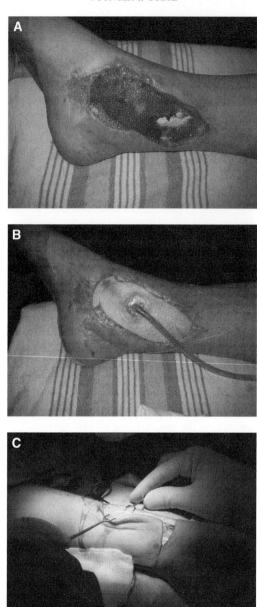

Fig. 8. A patient with an old gunshot wound to the medial malleolus associated with a medial malleolar nonunion and split skin graft presented with osteomyelitis and skin breakdown. (*A*) After debridement the posterior tibial tendon was exposed. The posterior tibial artery was compromised by atherosclerosis. Vascular bypass was required before free flap coverage. (*B*) In the interim, a VAC dressing was used to keep the wound clean. (*C*) A radial forearm flap suitable for such a defect was harvested.

compromised recipient beds. The disadvantages include donor site morbidity, increased operative time, and technical difficulty. Complications and failure rates are similar to those seen with local flaps [37].

Selection of free flap

Factors that are involved in selection of a particular flap include the defect size. A deep defect or void can be filled best by a muscle flap; however, a defect that requires bone to achieve fusion requires a bone composite free flap.

If contour is important, fascial or fasciocutaneous flaps are preferable. Patient positioning may limit or make the harvesting of a flap difficult. For example, the scapular flap requires the patient to be in the lateral or prone position. An adequate pedicle length is required to avoid the inconvenience, added operative time, and risk for vein grafting. A longer pedicle allows greater freedom for flap insetting, and the anastomosis can be moved out of a zone of injury (Fig. 8).

Each surgeon is familiar with a subset of flaps that makes ease of harvest, insertion, and donor defect closure safer and faster. Free flaps have been described in detail elsewhere [26,38].

Postoperative care

Immobilization or bed rest is maintained for a minimum 5 days after local or free flap coverage procedures. Dressing changes are performed at 5 to 7 days, and progressive gravity stress is commenced. Compression stockings can be worn beginning at 2 weeks and are helpful out to 6 months in controlling edema. Weight bearing can be commenced at 6 weeks if the underlying reconstruction allows.

Postoperative monitoring by temperature, or Doppler or laser Doppler probe is used for free flaps. The first 24 to 72 hours are the critical period for the flap. The authors monitor the flap for 5 days and keep the patient on a continuous infusion of IV dextran and oral aspirin.

Summary

Posttraumatic foot and ankle reconstruction requires careful preoperative planning to reduce wound complications. Systemic and local factors need to be considered. A careful surgical technique can avoid the need for surgical soft tissue coverage. Recognition of the need for coverage preoperatively improves outcomes. Often, dressings and time allow minor wound complications to heal. More severe wound issues require early soft tissue coverage by local or free flaps to prevent failure of the surgery.

References

[1] Godina M. Early microsurgical reconstruction of complex trauma of the extremities. Plast Reconstr Surg 1986;78(3):285–92.

[2] Armstrong DG, Lavery LA, Abu-Rumman P, et al. Outcomes of subatmospheric pressure dressing therapy on wounds of the diabetic foot. Ostomy Wound Manage 2002;48(4): 64–8.

[3] Berg E, Barth E, Clarke D, et al. The use of adjunctive hyperbaric oxygen in treatment of orthopedic infections and problem wounds: an overview and case reports. J Invest Surg 1989; 2(4):409–21.

[4] Lassen NA, Tonnesen KH, Holstein P. Distal blood pressure. Scand J Clin Lab Invest 1976; 36:705–9.

[5] Holstein P, Noer I, Thomasen KH. Distal blood pressure in severe arterial insufficiency. In: Began J, Yao J, editors. Gangrene and severe ischaemia in the lower extremities. New York: Grune and Stratton; 1978.

[6] Giordano CP, Koval KJ. Treatment of fracture blisters: a prospective study of 53 cases. J Orthop Trauma 1995;9(2):171–6.

[7] Attinger C, Cooper P. Soft tissue reconstruction for calcaneal fractures or osteomyelitis. Orthop Clin North Am 2001;32(1):135–70.

[8] Eginton MT, Brown KR, Seabrook GR, et al. A prospective randomized evaluation of negative-pressure wound dressings for diabetic foot wounds. Ann Vasc Surg 2003;17(6):645–9.

[9] Mantey I, Foster AV, Spencer S, et al. Why do foot ulcers recur in diabetic patients? Diabet Med 1999;16(3):245–9.

[10] Connor H, Mahdi OZ. Repetitive ulceration in neuropathic patients. Diabetes Metab Res Rev 2004;20(Suppl 1):S23–8.

[11] Attinger C, Cooper P, Blume P, et al. The safest surgical incisions and amputations applying the angiosome principles and using the Doppler to assess the arterial-arterial connections of the foot and ankle. Foot Ankle Clin 2001;6(4):745–99.

[12] Freiman A, Bird G, Metelitsa AI, et al. Cutaneous effects of smoking. J Cutan Med Surg 2004; 8(6):415–23.

[13] Ciaravino ME, Friedell ML, Kammerlocher TC. Is hyperbaric oxygen a useful adjunct in the management of problem lower extremity wounds? Ann Vasc Surg 1996;10(6):558–62.

[14] Apelqvist J, Ragnarson-Tennvall G. Cavity foot ulcers in diabetic patients: a comparative study of cadexomer iodine ointment and standard treatment. An economic analysis alongside a clinical trial. Acta Derm Venereol 1996;76(3):231–5.

[15] Attinger CE, Bulan EJ. Debridement. The key initial first step in wound healing. Foot Ankle Clin 2001;6(4):627–60.

[16] Josty IC, Ramaswamy R, Laing JH. Vacuum assisted closure: an alternative strategy in the management of degloving injuries of the foot. Br J Plast Surg 2001;54(4):363–5.

[17] Clare MP, Fitzgibbons TC, McMullen ST, et al. Experience with the vacuum assisted closure negative pressure technique in the treatment of non-healing diabetic and dysvascular wounds. Foot Ankle Int 2002;23(10):896–901.

[18] McCallon SK, Knight CA, Valiulus JP, et al. Vacuum-assisted closure versus saline-moistened gauze in the healing of postoperative diabetic foot wounds. Ostomy Wound Manage 2000;46(8): 28–32, 34.

[19] Espensen EH, Nixon BP, Lavery LA, et al. Use of subatmospheric (VAC) therapy to improve bioengineered tissue grafting in diabetic foot wounds. J Am Podiatr Med Assoc 2002;92(7): 395–7.

[20] Mazzucco L, Medici D, Serra M, et al. The use of autologous platelet gel to treat difficult-to-heal wounds: a pilot study. Transfusion 2004;44(7):1013–8.

[21] Crovetti G, Martinelli G, Issi M, et al. Platelet gel for healing cutaneous chronic wounds. Transfus Apher Sci 2004;30(2):145–51.

[22] Herouy Y, Mellios P, Bandemir E, et al. Autologous platelet-derived wound healing factor

promotes angiogenesis via alphavbeta3-integrin expression in chronic wounds. Int J Mol Med 2000;6(5):515–9.

[23] Niinikoski JH. Clinical hyperbaric oxygen therapy, wound perfusion, and transcutaneous oximetry. World J Surg 2004;28(3):307–11.

[24] Hudson DA, Millar K. The cross-leg flap: still a useful flap in children. Br J Plast Surg 1992;45(2):146–9.

[25] Attinger CE, Ducic I, Cooper P, et al. The role of intrinsic muscle flaps of the foot for bone coverage in foot and ankle defects in diabetic and nondiabetic patients. Plast Reconstr Surg 2002;110(4):1047–54 [discussion 55–7].

[26] Baumeister S, Germann G. Soft tissue coverage of the extremely traumatized foot and ankle. Foot Ankle Clin 2001;6(4):867–903.

[27] Hammert WC, Minarchek J, Trzeciak MA. Free-flap reconstruction of traumatic lower extremity wounds. Am J Orthop 2000;29(9 Suppl):22–6.

[28] Brunelli GA, Brunelli F, Brunelli GR. Microsurgical reconstruction of sensory skin. Ann Acad Med Singapore 1995;24(4 Suppl):108–12.

[29] Hallock GG, Rice DC, Keblish PA, et al. Restoration of the foot using the radial forearm flap. Ann Plast Surg 1988;20(1):14–25.

[30] Goldberg JA, Adkins PT, Sai TM. Microvascular reconstruction of the foot: weight-bearing patterns, gait analysis, and long-term follow-up. Plast Reconstr Surg 1993;92(5):904–11.

[31] Hermanson A, Dalsgaard CJ, Arnander C, et al. Sensibility and cutaneous reinnervation in free flaps. Plast Reconstr Surg 1987;79(3):422–7.

[32] Heinz T. Local flaps for hind foot reconstruction. Oper Tech Plastic Reconstr Surg 1997;4(4): 157–64.

[33] Attinger C. Soft-tissue coverage for lower-extremity trauma. Orthop Clin North Am 1995; 26(2):295–334.

[34] Hasegawa M, Torii S, Katoh H, et al. The distally based superficial sural artery flap. Plast Reconstr Surg 1994;93(5):1012–20.

[35] Masquelet AC, Romana MC, Wolf G. Skin island flaps supplied by the vascular axis of the sensitive superficial nerves: anatomic study and clinical experience in the leg. Plast Reconstr Surg 1992;89(6):1115–21.

[36] Leitner DW, Gordon L, Buncke HJ. The extensor digitorum brevis as a muscle island flap. Plast Reconstr Surg 1985;76(5):777–80.

[37] Serafin D, Georgiade NG, Smith DH. Comparison of free flaps with pedicled flaps for coverage of defects of the leg or foot. Plast Reconstr Surg 1977;59(4):492–9.

[38] Ferreira MC, Besteiro JM, Monteiro Jr AA, et al. Reconstruction of the foot with microvascular free flaps. Microsurgery 1994;15(1):33–6.

ELSEVIER
SAUNDERS

Foot Ankle Clin N Am
11 (2006) 237–251

FOOT AND
ANKLE CLINICS

Index

Note: Page numbers of article titles are in **boldface** type.

1083-7515/06/$ – see front matter © 2006 Elsevier Inc. All rights reserved.
doi:10.1016/S1083-7515(06)00015-5

Changing Your Address?

Make sure your subscription changes too! When you notify us of your new address, you can help make our job easier by including an exact copy of your Clinics label number with your old address (see illustration below.) This number identifies you to our computer system and will speed the processing of your address change. Please be sure this label number accompanies your old address and your corrected address—you can send an old Clinics label with your number on it or just copy it exactly and send it to the address listed below.

We appreciate your help in our attempt to give you continuous coverage. Thank you.

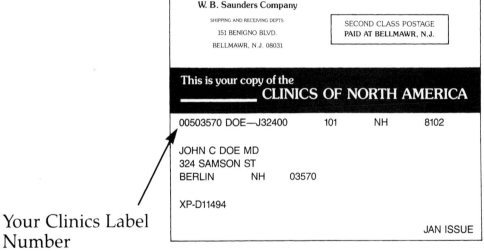

W. B. Saunders Company
SHIPPING AND RECEIVING DEPTS.
151 BENIGNO BLVD.
BELLMAWR, N.J. 08031

SECOND CLASS POSTAGE
PAID AT BELLMAWR, N.J.

This is your copy of the
_____ CLINICS OF NORTH AMERICA

00503570 DOE—J32400   101   NH   8102

JOHN C DOE MD
324 SAMSON ST
BERLIN   NH   03570

XP-D11494

JAN ISSUE

Your Clinics Label Number
Copy it exactly or send your label
along with your address to:
W.B. Saunders Company, Customer Service
Orlando, FL 32887-4800
Call Toll Free 1-800-654-2452

Please allow four to six weeks for delivery of new subscriptions and for processing address changes.